Gynae Geek

Gynae Geek

Your no-nonsense guide to
'down-there' healthcare

Dr Anita Mitra

Thorsons

Thorsons
An imprint of
HarperCollins*Publishers*
1 London Bridge Street
London SE1 9GF

www.harpercollins.co.uk

First published by HarperCollins*Publishers* 2019

1 3 5 7 9 10 8 6 4 2

Text © Dr Anita Mitra 2019

Illustrations © Nicolette Caven 2019

Dr Anita Mitra asserts the moral right to be
identified as the author of this work

A catalogue record of this book is available
from the British Library

ISBN 978-0-00-830517-8

Printed and bound in Great Britain by
CPI Group (UK) Ltd, Croydon, CR0 4YY

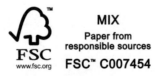

MIX
**Paper from
responsible sources**
FSC™ C007454
www.fsc.org

This book is produced from independently certified FSC paper
to ensure responsible forest management.

For more information visit: www.harpercollins.co.uk/green

For Menelaos, Achini and my mum

Contents

Acknowledgements

It is such an honour to write something for the whole world to see. But I couldn't have done it without the support of some incredible human beings who deserve huge thanks.

To Dr Rupy Aujla, my brother from another mother, for being the one who forced me to put myself out there to talk about something I believe the world needs to know.

To Dr Laura Thomas, for taking a chance on *The Gynae Geek* and inviting me on her podcast to discuss vaginas before that was a 'cool' thing to do.

To Dr Hazel Wallace and Alice Liveing, who both gave me a massive leg-up by collaborating with me on their social-media channels and giving me valuable advice about how to survive in the online world.

To Carly Cook, for her sass and support throughout the book-writing process and for hydrating me with many a mint tea. To the wonderful HarperCollins team – Carolyn Thorne, who saw the potential in my idea, George Atsiaris, Josie Turner and Julie McBrayne, who brought the campaign to life – thank you all!

To Adam Willis, my strength coach, but most of all my friend, for always being a voice of reason.

To my best friend, Achini Wanasinghe, and my mum, who listen to my moaning on a daily basis and support me no matter what. And all my other friends who have put up with being ignored for the time that I've spent writing the book.

To both of my parents for giving me the education that enabled me to be in the position to write this book.

To all the patients and my social-media followers who shared their stories and asked the questions that inspired it.

And finally, to Menelaos Tzafetas, aka 'Mr Gynae Geek', for being the one, in so many ways.

Introduction: Down-there healthcare by the Gynae Geek

It's three o'clock on a Wednesday afternoon and I've just performed a surgical evacuation on a woman who was nine weeks pregnant before she miscarried. I'm in theatre, writing an operation note, when my bleep goes off. It's A&E. I speak to a worried-sounding nurse who asks me to come urgently and see a patient: 'Forty-one years old ... bleeding very heavily . . . not pregnant . . . haemoglobin is four and—'

'What did you say? FOUR?' I jump in.

'Yes, Doctor, four—'

'OK, I'm coming. Put her in resus. And put in a large cannula if you don't already have good IV access. Oh, and what is her pulse?'

'One hundred and seven.'

'OK, I'm coming, I'm coming.'

I'm worried. Why is this patient's haemoglobin level almost one third of what is normal for a healthy female? I scrawl the rest of my notes in my best 'I'm-in-a-rush-but-I'm-trying-to-make-this-as-legible-as-possible' handwriting, a skill that's almost second nature now. I grab a disposable green paper gown to cover my theatre scrubs and run down the corridor to A&E. I enter the resus department, my gown fanning out rather dramatically behind me, and rush into the patient's cubicle.

She is hooked up to a machine that is beeping wildly because of her racing pulse, and there is a lot of blood on the bed. The nurse I spoke to on the phone looks concerned, standing over the patient who seems surprisingly calm, albeit slightly clammy. I ask her if she's sure she isn't pregnant; she laughs and tells me it's impossible, and the nurse confirms the pregnancy test is negative. She tells me she's having her period, but it's much heavier than normal. I ask her how many pads she's been using.

'Pads?' she asks. 'Oh, I don't use those until Day 2 or 3 when things have settled down. I normally take the first day or two off work and sit on folded-up bath towels because there's so much bleeding. Today it was so heavy though that I was just sat in the shower for a few hours, washing away the blood as it came out. But I didn't feel well, and I think I might have passed out, so I called an ambulance.'

I look at the patient, who is slightly obese and of South Asian descent, which, along with her symptoms, makes me begin to suspect she has a cancer. I ask her how long she's had this bleeding.

'Probably about twenty years.'

Twenty. Years. No wonder her haemoglobin is four. In fact, I'm surprised she made it this far without ever having had to come to hospital, especially as she has been losing iron at the speed of sound for two decades.

I perform an internal examination and blood clots the size of my palm begin to fall out of her vagina. Then, miraculously, the bleeding seems to stop. I wait for a few seconds to see if more blood will come out. Nothing. I wait some more . . . and some more . . . and then there's another steady trickle. I instruct the nurse to get me some IV tranexamic acid (a drug to stop bleeding) urgently, which she does, and I administer it myself. I prescribe a blood transfusion and tell the nurse to give some IV fluids to stabilise the patient, while we wait for the blood to be cross-matched in the lab. I also prescribe tablets to slow down the bleeding.

As I wait to give the tranexamic acid time to work, I ask the patient – trying not to sound patronising – why she has never sought help for her heavy periods. She tells me she had come to think it was normal, and even a few years ago when she began to suspect it was not, she was too embarrassed to discuss it with friends or family, or to go and speak to her GP. As we talk, her bleeding slows down, and I arrange for her to be transferred to the gynaecology ward. She will be observed and receive a blood transfusion, though I have no idea at this point that she will need four units of blood.

Walking away from A&E, I can't believe what I have just seen. And I realise I will never get over the shock I feel when patients drop this kind of bombshell; nor will I ever truly understand the extraordinary things some people accept as 'normal'.

*   *   *

If you're still with me, and are not feeling too queasy from my casual Wednesday-afternoon bloodbath, let me introduce myself. My name is Dr Anita Mitra, B.Sc., M.B.Ch.B., Ph.D. I'm a London-based doctor, qualified in 2011 and I'm now training to be a specialist in Obstetrics and Gynaecology (O&G). I have almost fifteen years of clinical and lab-based research experience under the belt of my oversized NHS tie-top scrubs. An interesting fact is that my surname is the Greek word for 'uterus' – although I'm not actually Greek, and I didn't always want to be a gynaecologist.

Now sit tight if you're ready to hear the somewhat off-piste route that led me to become the turmeric-latte loving, dead-lifting doctor who removes disco balls from 'you-know-where' for a living . . .

From the age of about three, I wanted to follow in my father's footsteps and become a surgeon. But at seventeen, I was far too cool for school and, as a result, the only A grade I got in my A-levels was in German, which didn't do much for any of the medical schools I'd applied to. I ended up talking my way into a place on a Medical Biochemistry course at the University of Leicester, after the admissions tutor told me my grades were 'a bit lower' than they'd normally accept. During my time reading Medical Biochemistry I worked in a research lab, studying the anticancer mechanisms of plant-based chemicals (which is essentially the scientific basis for the current turmeric latte trend). This was the first time I truly appreciated the impact of diet and lifestyle on our health. I worked my socks off during my undergraduate years and graduated three years later with a first-class degree and a place at Leicester Medical School.

For the first few years of medical school, I still desperately wanted to be a surgeon, and spent the third and fourth years doing research in my spare time with a professor of kidney-transplant surgery. However, in my fifth year, I had to do my placement in Obstetrics & Gynaecology. I have to admit I was partly terrified and partly bored by the idea of spending eight weeks in the speciality. However, those eight weeks changed my life. I loved the interaction with the patients, both young and old, the diseases fascinated me and the surgery was often bloody and dramatic, but usually with great outcomes, which I loved. Suddenly, I knew this was exactly what I wanted to do for the rest of my life.

I graduated from medical school in the summer of 2011 and spent my first two years working as a doctor in the East Midlands, completing the mandatory Foundation Programme, which involves basic training in six different specialties. My first job was, in fact, in Obstetrics & Gynaecology, and it flew by in an adrenaline-fuelled, placenta-splattered blur. I had found my calling. But it wasn't plain sailing from there. I wanted to move to London and O&G training was very competitive at the time, with nine applicants for every job, and unfortunately, I didn't get one. There is only one chance to apply annually, so I needed to find something else to do for a year. Many doctors work as locums, filling gaps on rotas for very good money, but I have never been driven by cash, and after my initial disappointment, I saw this year as an opportunity to enrich myself and my CV.

Failure always feeds my hunger, but I needed to ensure that failure was not an option with my next chance at a training job. So to cut a very long story short, I decided that I would still try and move to London and pursue my love of research for a year. To make this happen, my plan was to email every single professor of Obstetrics & Gynaecology in London and beg them for a research job. And it worked! I got a prestigious position at Imperial College, London, where I started doing a Ph.D. – the most incredible, but challenging thing I've ever done. And during that time, I managed to bag myself one of those sought-after training jobs.

As much as I thrive on the thrill of operating and the honour of being able to help women bring their babies into the world, the thing I love most about my job is the chance to sit down with them to answer their questions about gynaecological health and calm their anxieties. Many concerns often stem from lack of knowledge and understanding of what is 'normal' – because very few women feel it is safe to talk about a topic shrouded in taboos and shame. While there is so much general health information available online, there is relatively little engaging and reliable material about female health. There are also lots of unqualified people selling their opinions as medical fact. I began to see the conversation opening up on social media, but when I looked closer it filled me with horror. Film stars talking about vaginal steaming, beauty bloggers talking about vaginal facials, wellness coaches telling women they had successfully 'detoxed their body' because their vegan diet had stopped their periods, as well as other unqualified people pushing products that women simply don't need. But where were all the doctors?

Women drink in this information, unable to decide for themselves whether it is actually credible or evidence-based, distracted by the huge numbers of followers these 'experts' have and the glossy façade of the online world.

I saw the need for a sensible voice in this unregulated chaos, so I started an online blog and Instagram account called 'Gynae Geek'. The positive response was overwhelming. I began to receive huge numbers of comments and messages from women desperate to know more, and I get a particular thrill from seeing them tagging their friends in my posts for them to read.

I realise that I am in a privileged position, with over fifteen years of scientific and clinical training that have given me the ability to seek out information and decide whether it is credible or not. This is one of the reasons that I back up most posts with references to scientific studies – to prove to my followers that what I'm providing them with is reliable information and not just my opinion. It is also why I use the word 'geek': I want women to realise that knowledge is sexy, knowledge is power and that they should never be afraid to ask: 'Why?' and 'How?'

So, what is this book about?

This is not your average healthcare book. While it's full of medical and scientific facts, it's also a collection of tales from the thousands of patients I've treated, who inspired many of the topics in the book. It is a back-to-basics guide to gynae-cological health, covering what's normal and what's not. It's sensible, no-nonsense and, most of all, evidence-based. Some parts might make you blush, others make you laugh and some might even make you exclaim, 'Oh my gosh, that's me!' But it's not intended for self-diagnosis, nor as an alter-native to visiting a doctor in real life. Rather, it is designed to help you to decide whether or not you need to go and talk to a healthcare professional about something that's bother-ing you.

I also hope this book will be a conversation starter for women of all ages – because we need to break the taboo around talking about what's going on down there. The reluc-tance to do so often delays women in seeking the help they need, which can result in unnecessary suffering and poor health outcomes. I want women to see that there is no ques-tion that cannot be asked, no symptom that should be ignored and, most importantly, no need to suffer if they are in need of help.

As well as covering anatomy and the mechanics, sexual health and fertility, I've also included a section on lifestyle and women's wellbeing, which form one of my favourite sub-jects. A lot of women do not realise there is a link between gynaecological health and how we eat, sleep, move and gen-erally live our lives. There are a surprising number of simple things that can be done on a daily basis to help you and your health today and for the future.

Each chapter includes a section headed 'Things you've always wanted to know, but were too afraid to ask' – a col-lection of questions I'm most frequently asked in relation to the particular topic in hand. The chapters then conclude with a short summary – 'The Gynae Geek's knowledge bombs'

– which comprises the essentials that everyone should take away from the chapter.

*　*　*

I set out to write a book that would be engaging and entertaining at times (the opposite of most of the health information that is out there at the moment). And while there are areas where I've shared my opinion, as a scientist and a doctor I have been insistent that the information provided is evidence-based and that's why you'll see so many references everywhere.

The structure and content have been led by questions my patients, friends and social-media followers have asked me. You may decide to skip over certain sections because they don't apply to you at the moment. But they may do in the future. Or they may apply to your friend/sister/colleague right now – and I would be honoured if you would share this book with other women who you think would benefit. But also share it with the men in your lives. Because women's health shouldn't be a mystery to them either. The health of the nation depends on the health of its women and, therefore, it's something that everyone should be aware of.

My ultimate goal with this book is to ensure that every woman has access to the information she needs to understand how her body works, to empower her to seek help and thus ensure that no one suffers in silence.

Now go forth, learn, enjoy and don't ever forget that it's cool to be a geek!

PART ONE

Anatomy

Since we're just getting to know one another, I want to share a fact about myself: I'm quite good at charades. Why is that? Because most people seem to use hand gestures, rather than actual words when it comes to their vagina/undercarriage/'down there'/lady garden/private parts – whatever you want to call it. The fact is, most women I encounter don't know the proper names for their genitalia. And some wince when I say the word V.A.G.I.N.A. But I want to shout it from the rooftops. It's not a dirty word! And I think this difficulty with using the right language is one of the major reasons why people feel embarrassed to go and see a doctor when they're concerned something is not right: because they don't even know what to call the area in question. That's why this section provides you with an informal anatomy lesson, with a few interesting anecdotes along the way. So don't be shy, it's time to learn the essentials.

CHAPTER 1

External female genital anatomy

Doctor, while you're down there, can you just tell me if my vagina looks normal?

This is one of the questions I am most frequently asked by my patients, but it is also one of the most inaccurately phrased. What women actually mean is: 'Does my vulva look normal?'

Many people don't know the difference between the vulva and vagina, and I think this is a major reason why women so often feel embarrassed to go and see a doctor when they're concerned that something is not right: because they don't even know what to call the area they are worried about. What's more, women's perceptions of a 'normal vulva' are usually inaccurately shaped by the pornography industry, and as someone who looks at vulvas (and vaginas) for a living, I feel appropriately qualified to suggest that this area is becoming a target for body dysmorphia.

It's very common for women to feel embarrassed or ashamed to take their clothes off and a lot of women apologise as I begin an examination, but it's important to remember that, as awkward as it may make you feel as a patient, as healthcare professionals we're totally relaxed and at home. So with that out of the way, let me take you on a brief tour of your anatomy.

The vulva

Vulva, a word that makes a lot of people giggle or blush, is the term used to refer to the external genital region containing the following structures:

- **Mons pubis** Also known as the Mound of Venus, this is the fatty tissue that covers the front of the pubic bone and is covered in hair. A lot of women apologise for not shaving or waxing this area, but there is no evidence to show that hair removal improves hygiene or reduces the risk of infections, so you don't actually need to (see page 6 for more on this). Pubic hair also plays a protective role in cushioning the sensitive underlying skin, as well as collecting pheromones, the chemicals that play a role in sexual attraction.

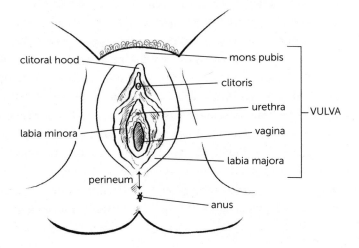

- **Clitoris and clitoral hood** Your clitoris is shaped like the wishbone of a chicken. The clitoral head, about the size of a small pea, is the visible part of the clitoris, but is, in fact, just the tip of the iceberg, because extending down either side underneath the skin are two arms, each about 5–7cm long. The clitoris is made of the same kind of spongy tissue that is found in the centre of a penis, which fills with blood to produce an erection, and the same thing happens to the clitoris during arousal. The clitoral head has the same embryological origin as the head of the penis but contains about two to three times as many nerves, and might explain why it doesn't need to be pressed like a doorbell with a dead battery, which many men don't realise. The sensitive nature is also the reason that there is a fold of skin usually covering it, called the clitoral hood.
- **Urethral opening** The urethra is the tube that empties urine from the bladder. It's much shorter in women, at only about 5cm, compared to 20cm in men, which is why women are more likely to get urinary tract infections (UTIs). This is also the reason why you should wipe front to back after using the toilet, and urinate after sex in order to avoid helping the spread of bacteria into the urethra and up into the bladder. Some women may be able to see their urethral opening, while others cannot, and that's because it can be quite high up, sometimes even almost inside the vagina. I've seen many a medical student try to put a catheter into the clitoris, but it's always the boys who blush the most when I politely redirect them to the urethra!
- **Periurethral/Skene's glands** I've often been asked at parties by overexcited men about female ejaculation. Well, these are the glands that are responsible for this

phenomenon, and they are the female version of the prostate gland. The fluid they make is thought to offer some protection against the bugs that cause UTIs. Infrequently, they can get blocked and swell up, causing a cyst, which can sometimes be confused with a vaginal-wall prolapse.

○ **Vagina** This refers to the muscular tube inside that goes from your vaginal opening on the outside, up to the cervix. Your vagina cannot be seen from the outside (hence the inaccuracy of the question: 'Does my vagina look normal?'), and at about 7–9cm long, it has an amazing degree of elasticity and can expand in all directions – enough to allow for the birth of a baby. Its expansive nature also means it can also accommodate many a foreign object.

Possibly the most unusual thing I've ever removed from someone's vagina was a disco ball. Not a massive one from the ceiling of a 70s club, but one that was golf-ball-sized and originally belonged on a key chain. It was 7 a.m., and the end of a particularly harrowing night shift in A&E, but having been told that the offending object was a key ring, I thought it would be a quick job. Then the triage nurse casually added: 'Oh, by the way, Doc, the key ring itself has snapped off and it's just the disco ball left inside now . . . ' Needless to say, it certainly was a challenge, largely due to the fact that your vagina can make a pretty impressive vacuum, but I got it out in the end. If the owner of said disco ball is reading this, I just want to say how much I still feel your pain and embarrassment to this very day.

○ **Labia majora** These are the larger, skin-covered outer lips of the vulva. The skin here is usually darker than the rest of the surrounding skin and has a fatty layer underneath that plays a protective role.

- **Labia minora** These are the inner, more fleshy-looking lips, that are usually quite red or pink and probably what cause the most concern with regards to what's 'normal'. Most women's labia minora will be visible below the labia majora and it's common for them to be asymmetrical. The average size ranges from 2–10cm in length and 1–5cm in width[1] and consequently the appearance of the labia minora varies significantly from one woman to the next. It's kind of ironic how teenage boys (and let's be honest, most immature men) boast about the size of their penis, yet women are expected to have neat, tucked-in labia that never see the light of day. Why is this? Because they originate from the same embryological structure. It is normal for them to seem to enlarge slightly with age due to loss of collagen and oestrogen, both of which support the structure of the tissue.
- **Perineum** This is the area between the back of the vaginal opening and the anus.
- **Pelvic-floor muscles** Your pelvic floor is underneath the skin of the perineum and is made up of several muscles and pieces of connective tissue that act as a sling to hold your insides in. Pelvic-floor weakness can lead to prolapse of the vaginal walls, bladder, urethra or the uterus. A lot of people think you can only get a prolapse if you've had a baby, or if you've had a vaginal delivery, during which these muscles may tear or be cut to facilitate delivery. However, this is not the case, and it can happen to anyone – regardless of whether they've only ever had C-sections, or even if they've never had a baby. The pelvic-floor muscles also help you to maintain control of your bladder and bowel.

||||||||||||||||||||||||||||||||||||||||

THINGS YOU'VE ALWAYS WANTED TO KNOW, BUT WERE TOO AFRAID TO ASK

Is 'down-there' hair removal safe?

Generally speaking, yes. Minor cuts, burns and ingrown hairs may occur as a result, but they're rarely severe enough to require medical attention. The most commonly reported reason given for removing pubic hair is for hygiene purposes,[2] however there isn't actually any evidence to show that it improves hygiene or reduces the risk of infections. I think this belief is perpetuated by the myth that your vulva and vagina are dirty and teeming with germs. As doctors, we don't judge or have a preference about the terrain down there, so don't feel you have to schedule a waxing/shaving session before an appointment. I'll take it as it comes, thank you!

Will having lots of sex make my vagina loose?

No. Regardless of what the teenage boys in the playground may have said, this is not true. Your vagina is very elastic and can expand enough to let a baby out (and other objects in) but it always shrinks back. While having a baby may change the shape of your vagina slightly, having sex will not because a penis is not large enough to do so. Having sex will also not change the size or shape of your labia minora.

Do I need a labiaplasty?

Absolutely not! Labiaplasty is surgery to trim the labia minora and/or clitoral hood. It is largely performed for cosmetic reasons. I think that the sudden interest in 'neatening up' one's labia may be an undesirable offshoot of the current obsession with aesthetic 'perfection'. There are numerous plastic surgeons around the world advertising labiaplasty as a quick and simple procedure to make your labia more symmetrical/ neat and tidy, etc. But symmetry is overrated – no other body part is truly symmetrical: we've all got one foot that's bigger than the other, eyebrows that don't match. And it's the same with labia. It's also normal for your labia minora to be visible on the outside, although Barbie and the porn industry may tell you otherwise. There is minimal evidence to show that the surgery actually improves pain, sexual function or how women feel about their genitalia, plus there is a risk of pain after the surgery due to nerve damage or resulting scar tissue, so it's really not a decision to take lightly. And it cannot be reversed in the same way that you could, for example, have breast implants removed. As a famous professor once pointed out: 'If you think your labia are too long, stop shaving off your pubic hair and you're unlikely to think so.'

When should I start doing pelvic-floor exercises?

Right about . . . now! Also called Kegel exercises (see pages 217–18), everyone should be doing them, regardless of whether they are pregnant or have ever had a baby, because that's not the only thing that weakens them. They generally weaken with age, so you want them to be as strong as possible from a young age. Doing pelvic-floor exercises in pregnancy, especially from an early stage, has also been shown to reduce the amount of time it takes to push your baby out, and the risk of leaking urine after the birth.[3,4] Many people think having a Caesarean section prevents pelvic-floor weakness, but that's not the case. Carrying around several kilos of extra weight for nine months will put extra strain on the pelvic floor whether you push out that watermelon or it comes out the sunroof!

| | | | | | | | | | | | | | | | | | | | | | | | | | | | | | | | | | | | | | | | | |

THE GYNAE GEEK'S KNOWLEDGE BOMBS

The female vulva can generate a great deal of anxiety, but I hope you now feel more comfortable with describing the different areas should you ever need to talk to a doctor about it.

The following are the key facts that I would like you to take away from this chapter:

- Your vulva is on the outside; your vagina is on the inside.
- Your vulva looks normal. Don't let anyone tell you otherwise.
- Pubic hair removal is safe but doesn't carry any health benefits, so don't feel you have to do it.
- You do not need a labiaplasty if it's purely for appearance reasons. It's normal for your labia minora to hang below the labia majora and for one to be longer than the other. It's Barbie who got that part wrong, not you.
- Your pelvic-floor muscles are the lifelong friends that you need to get to know. Kegel exercises (see pages 217–18) are the most underrated workout that we should all be doing, not just in pregnancy.

CHAPTER 2

Internal female genital anatomy

(While I'm performing a vaginal examination
to look at a patient's cervix):
'Doctor, do my ovaries look healthy?'

To be clear, I can't see your ovaries when I'm looking up inside your vagina. Yet I've been asked this question on multiple occasions, which tells me that many women may need a refresher of that uninspiring biology class that we all sat through at school. I'll tell you about the cervix – what even is that? And a cervical ectropion, which is actually very common and completely healthy, yet one of the most anxiety-provoking things that I find myself explaining again and again. I'll also tell you about a few of the interesting lumps and bumps that I spend a lot of time talking about in clinic that can cause a lot of confusion, usually made worse by my rogue friend Dr Google.

The uterus

The uterus is also known as the womb, and we often use the terms interchangeably. I'll use the word uterus from now on, you know, in the name of being proper and all.

The uterus is a muscular structure found in your pelvis, behind your bladder and in front of your bowel. It's roughly pear-shaped, although I often describe it to patients as an upside-down wine bottle, with the large part of the bottle representing the body of the uterus and the neck representing the cervix (or neck of the womb), which acts as a passage for sperm to enter the uterus and menstrual blood or babies to exit. The wall of the uterus is made of smooth muscle, which moves in a ripple-type motion as opposed to striated muscle, which is the type you flex on demand in the gym. You might think that your uterus only contracts during labour, and while this may be the time when it performs its most vigorous workout, it also contracts during your period, helping the menstrual blood to escape, and during female orgasm. Given that these contractions are what cause you to have period pain, it's not unusual for some women to experience a similar kind of pain for a few hours after sex, either due to orgasm-induced contractions or just because their uterus actually gets a bit irritated from being poked about.

Endometrium

The endometrium is the lining of the uterus, and is at its thinnest around your period, gradually thickening throughout the month to make a nice, soft, juicy landing for a fertilised egg. If this doesn't happen, the lining is shed when you have your period. The thickness of the lining at the end of the month will determine how heavy your period is, and also, to some extent, how painful it may be – because the more there is to shed, the more the muscle of your uterus may need to contract to help move it out through the cervix and down into the vagina.

The cervix

The cervix or 'the neck of the wine bottle' is the gatekeeper to the uterus. Not only does it have a mechanical function of keeping your uterus shut during pregnancy, it also has a pretty complex immune function. A large quantity of the vaginal discharge that you produce comes from the cervix. Discharge is clever and anxiety-provoking in equal measures, which is why I have given it its own chapter (see Chapter 6). But until you get to that section, be aware that it's way more than just a lubricant and contains loads of 'natural antibiotics' that protect you against infections, and that changes in the texture and qualities of the discharge throughout the cycle can determine whether sperm is able to enter.

If you feel your cervix (for non-squeamish readers, this involves inserting your finger into your vagina and feeling right at the top), it usually feels like the tip of your nose, because there is a little indentation in the middle. This is called the 'external os' and is the entry into the cervical canal; the small tunnel that runs through the cervix up into the cavity of the uterus. The canal is usually only a couple of millimetres wide, but during labour it opens up to 10cm, which is what we call 'fully dilated'. Prostaglandins are the chemical messengers that cause contraction of your uterus during your period, and they also cause your cervix to soften slightly, opening a tiny bit to allow blood to escape with ease.

Cervical ectropion

An ectropion is an exposed area of the glandular lining of the inside of the cervix. Not everyone has one, but those who do are often terrified. And understandably so, because it is not

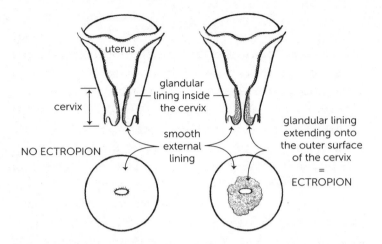

uterus

cervix

glandular
lining inside
the cervix

NO ECTROPION

smooth
external
lining

glandular lining
extending onto
the outer surface
of the cervix
=
ECTROPION

something that is usually described clearly. So let me give it a go . . . Normally, the outer cervix is covered entirely with a smooth lining that's quite tough and similar to the skin lining the inside of the vagina. But the glandular lining is a bit rough in texture, yet more fragile, and produces most of the protective discharge that I'll cover in Chapter 6. It's most common to have an ectropion when taking the combined oral contraceptive Pill, or during pregnancy, but loads of women just have one for no particular reason. They're not associated with a higher risk of abnormal smears, or with any other disease. They can be bloody annoying though – literally. They tend to bleed on contact, such as during a smear test or during/after sex due to the fragile nature of the glandular lining. It doesn't mean anything is wrong, it's just that the lining isn't really designed to be exposed in such a way.

Having said that, lots of women have an ectropion and never know because they don't all bleed. If you do have one it can go away on its own; especially if you're on the Pill it will often disappear when you stop taking it. But if the bleeding is really annoying, there are things that can be done to treat it, such as having the exposed glandular layer burned away, which is what a lot of websites will recommend. Many women come to clinic insisting they want it removed; we generally advise against it unless it's really problematic, and the vast majority change their mind once I've explained that it's not harmful. As one patient once said to me, 'If it's nothing sinister, I'll take a few harmless drops of blood over a barbecue on my cervix any day.'

Cervical polyps

These are little 'skin tags' that can be found in the cervix. Many women have them and never know, but in some they cause symptoms of abnormal discharge (a change in colour, texture, amount or bloodstained), bleeding in between periods, after sex or after a gynaecological examination, which makes them super annoying, and a potential source of worry. They may also be found by chance during a routine examination such as a smear test. They can be removed easily in clinic, and it's quick and painless, but if they're not causing symptoms this is unnecessary, as they are always benign (non-cancerous) and don't increase the risk of any kind of disease or trouble in the future.[5]

Nabothian follicle

Also called mucus-retention cyst, this is where the mucus that is made as part of the healthy function of the cervix becomes trapped underneath the surface of the cervix. Most often, these cysts are just an incidental finding when you're having a speculum examination, and they're usually too small to be felt, although if you touch your cervix, you may be able to feel the little lumps. They are completely normal and don't increase the risk of any kind of gynaecological disease, nor are they anything to do with sexually transmitted infections. A patient once told me that another doctor described them as spots/whiteheads on her cervix, and she had thought it was because she wasn't washing her vagina enough; so she went to town with various feminine-hygiene products, which didn't make them go away and just gave her terrible vaginal irritation. If you have them, you can't do anything to make them go away and you don't need to either.

Fallopian tubes

You have two fallopian tubes – one on the left and one on the right, coming off the top of your uterus like long ears that flap around and pick up eggs from the ovaries. I recently scanned a lady who was ecstatic to find out she was seven weeks pregnant. I showed her the pregnancy in the uterus with a heartbeat and told her I could see the egg had come from the left ovary. She looked baffled and said it wasn't possible because she'd had her left tube removed three years before due to an ectopic pregnancy (where the fertilised egg implants itself outside the uterus, usually in one of the tubes). However, your tubes are incredibly mobile – like a motorbike courier, they'll pick up from any location if the goods are ready and waiting. So even with one tube, eggs can still be picked up from either ovary. The tubes contain tiny little finger-like projections called cilia, which help to sweep the eggs along into the uterus. However, they are not directly attached to the ovaries, and open into the pelvic cavity, which can serve as a route for infections to spread from your vagina, which is how sexually transmitted infections in particular can spread and cause pelvic inflammatory disease (see Chapter 9).

Ovaries

You have two ovaries, which are held close to your uterus by two ligaments – one that attaches to the wall of the inside of your pelvis and one that attaches to your uterus. The ovaries are home to a woman's egg supply, which is complete at birth (about 2–4 million). The number of eggs decreases gradually as we age, with about three to five thousand ultimately making it to the point of being released. This is called ovulation and usually happens about once a month. The eggs live in little sacs called follicles, which go through several days of maturation to eventually form a cyst: a fluid-filled sac which bursts and releases an egg which may or may not then be fertilised.

Your ovaries are also a major site of hormone production, making the following:

○ **Oestrogens** Oestrogens, of which there are three types (oestrone, oestrodiol and oestriol), are not only responsible for your menstrual cycle, but also play a role in memory, heart health, bone strength and even the immune system.

○ **Progesterone** The major site of progesterone production is from the corpus luteum – this is the 'shell' that is left behind in the ovary after ovulation. If you don't ovulate, very little progesterone will come from the ovaries themselves and the adrenal glands. (These glands sit above your kidneys and are responsible for making small amounts of progesterone along with a whole host of other very important hormones.) Levels are highest seven days after ovulating – that is Day 21 if you have a twenty-eight-day cycle – so if you're having blood tests to see if you're ovulating, this is what will be checked. If your level is low, you either didn't ovulate or the timing of the test was wrong. The latter is surprisingly common, and a lot of scared patients come to clinic worried that they're not ovulating. On further questioning, they do describe all the signs of ovulation (see Chapter 3), and I'm then able to help them work out when to do the test, after which they come back very happy with a nice high progesterone reading.

○ **Inhibin** This hormone sends a message from the ovaries back to the brain saying, 'We're being stimulated enough, thanks'.

○ **Relaxin** This is a hormone which causes the joints and ligaments to soften during pregnancy to prepare the body for labour. It's also responsible for the joint pain that pregnant women often experience.

○ **Testosterone** This is usually associated with men, but believe it or not, women need it too – not just to promote sex drive, but also for bone and muscle strength, as well as brain function.

||||||||||||||||||||||||||||||||||||||||||||

THINGS YOU'VE ALWAYS WANTED TO KNOW, BUT WERE TOO AFRAID TO ASK

What is a retroverted uterus and will it affect my chances of getting pregnant?

Also known as a tipped/tilted uterus, it means the uterus points backwards (retroverted) instead of forwards (anteverted). Between 20 and 30 per cent of women have this and in many cases, it is just how they were born and bears no impact on their health. In some women, however, it may be due to conditions such as endometriosis (see pages 59–60), fibroids (see pages 57–8) or the presence of scar tissue that pulls the uterus backwards. The actual position of the uterus does not affect your chances of getting pregnant because sperm is able to swim in all directions; however, any one of the underlying conditions above may cause problems. It also doesn't cause pain, but again, if it's due to an underlying disease, that may do so.

A retroverted uterus can make your cervix a little trickier to find when you have a smear test, which can be slightly uncomfortable. But we know plenty of tricks to make it easier and less painful. I often use the 'make-fists-and-put-them-underneath-your-bottom' position – if you know, you know! But the smear itself shouldn't be any worse than normal.

As the uterus increases in size in pregnancy, it will gradually flip forward, and by twelve weeks – when most women are having their first scan – a retroverted uterus may have corrected itself, so that many women never even find out they had one.

Why do I bleed after sex?

Also called post-coital bleeding, bleeding after sex can have many causes, including:

○ cervical ectropion (see pages 11–13)
○ cervical and endometrial polyps (see page 13)
○ infections such as chlamydia, or even something simple like thrush, which causes irritation of the vagina and cervix and the added friction of sex can be enough to make it bleed
○ vaginal dryness (lack of lubrication, which can make the vaginal tissue more sensitive to friction in particular)
○ skin conditions such as psoriasis or lichen schlerosus – these can make the skin more delicate and increase the chance of getting small skin tears

- cervical cancer – the one that everyone worries about, but is actually the least likely cause, which is why I've put it at the bottom of the list; the risk ranges from 1 in 44,000 cases of post-coital bleeding in women aged 20–24 to 1 in 2,400 in 45–54-year-olds.[6]

Does removing a fallopian tube affect my fertility?

Sometimes fallopian tubes may need to be removed in cases of severe infections (see Chapter 9 on STIs) or due to an ectopic pregnancy (a pregnancy in the tube). You can still get pregnant with one tube (see page 14), but if both are removed it does mean that you would need IVF to get pregnant. Removing either one or both tubes also does not affect the function of your ovaries and does not cause you to go into the menopause.

Why do I have a cyst on my ovary?

Ovarian cysts are very common and about 1 in 10 women will need surgery for one at some point in their lifetime. Most arise as a result of the normal workings of the ovary (see pages 15–16). We get tonnes of referrals to the gynaecology clinic for ovarian cysts that have been found incidentally during a scan for something else. Ultrasound is the best way to look at your ovaries initially, preferably an internal scan using a small probe inside the vagina because it gets closer to the action. Most cysts will disappear on their own within a couple of months. You may need a follow-up ultrasound, depending on the size and type of cyst.

Larger cysts may need to be removed because there is a greater risk that they may twist the ovary which cuts off its blood supply, and if not untwisted will cause the ovary to die. This is called 'ovarian torsion', and you'll definitely know if you have it because it is incredibly painful, to the point where even morphine won't touch the pain. It requires emergency surgery to untwist the ovary and remove the cyst. In most cases the ovary itself can be saved if the blood supply returns on untwisting.

The biggest ovarian cyst I've ever seen was in a young woman and was 24cm across. She was supermodel-slim, and finally went to her GP after spending a fortune on pregnancy tests, because she couldn't understand why they were all negative, yet she looked seven months pregnant. A big tummy is a slightly unusual way for a cyst to present. More common symptoms include:

o abdominal pain – this may be constant, occasional or during sex
o constipation – due to pressure on your bowel
o wanting to pass urine more often – due to pressure on your bladder
o a change in your periods – irregular, heavier or lighter.
o The risk of a cyst being cancerous in a pre-menopausal woman is very low, ranging from 1 to 3 in 1000.[7] (See Chapter 4 for more about polycystic ovaries.)

Should I be worried about ovarian cancer?

Ovarian cancer is so rare before the menopause and ovarian cysts do not increase your risk.

An estimated 5–15 per cent of ovarian cancers are inherited, most often caused by mutations in the BRCA1 and 2 genes, which are also associated with breast cancers. If you have close family members (e.g. mother, sister, grandmother) affected by ovarian cancer, particularly at a young age, you may be eligible for genetic testing, which should be discussed with a genetic counsellor.

An estimated 21 per cent of cases of ovarian cancer are directly related to lifestyle factors including smoking, poor diet and lack of exercise,[8] so keeping active and eating well is one of the best ways to prevent the disease.

There isn't currently any screening for ovarian cancer, as there isn't yet a test that is accurate enough. Remember that screening means identifying women who may have a disease but do not have any symptoms.

If you experience any of the following symptoms more than twelve times per month, you should be investigated:

○ Persistent bloating
○ Feeling easily full after eating and/or loss of appetite
○ Pelvic or abdominal pain
○ Needing to pass urine more often, or as a matter of urgency
○ Change in bowel habit

|||||||||||||||||||||||||||||||||||||||

THE GYNAE GEEK'S KNOWLEDGE BOMBS

I hope you have found this chapter more fascinating than when you studied female anatomy in that awkward biology lesson at school. These are the key facts that you may not have learned back then that I want you to keep in mind:

o Your uterus can face forwards or backwards and contracts during your period to help the blood get out, which is what causes period pain.
o It also doesn't like being poked very much, which is why it can be normal to get a bit of an ache after sex.
o Bleeding after sex is rarely caused by the big C.
o Your fallopian tubes are pretty flexible guys, flapping around like a Mexican wave, so that they can pick up an egg from either ovary.
o Ovarian cysts are very common (often a result of the normal functioning of your ovary) and do not increase your risk of ovarian cancer.

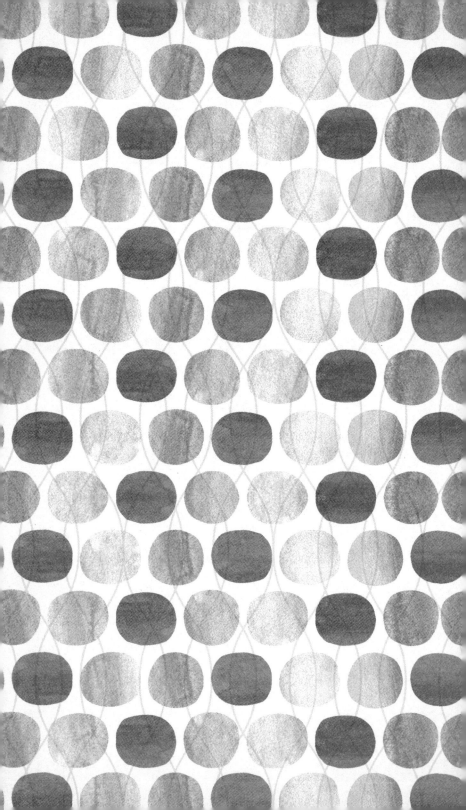

PART TWO

Periods

Periods are one of society's biggest taboos. Over half of the population has had or will have one at some point during their lifetime. Yet we barely talk about them.

I've noticed an interesting three-way split in the way women feel about periods. In the first group are women who are ambivalent; they don't mind either way whether they come or not. The second group hate them and would do anything to make them go away ('Give me anything you've got to make them stop!'). The third group love them and are horrified at the thought of not having their period every month – some, because they see it as a sign that their bodies are working, and many because they feel like it's 'cleaning their body from the inside' (although I'm always quite keen to point out that having a period doesn't clean your body of germs or toxins; in fact, I think period blood often has a 'dirty' connotation, which is probably one of the reasons we're so reluctant to address the issue).

There are some types of contraception – for example, the hormonal coil – that will stop your periods (see Chapter 7), and if that happens it's not a bad thing. It doesn't mean your uterus will become 'unclean'. The medication is simply preventing the lining from building up, so there's nothing to shed. I once offered the hormonal coil to a lady whose periods were so heavy that she'd had several blood transfusions. However, for her the possibility of having no period at all was unacceptable and she declined, explaining that she 'wouldn't feel like a woman any more'. I really like the fact that some women appreciate their period as a sign that their body is working. This is so true, and I always tell my patients that their period is a reflection of what's been going on in their bodies for the last month, even slightly longer.

The next three chapters will cover the basics of periods, the menstrual cycle and what can, and commonly does go wrong.

CHAPTER 3

Periods – the basics

Me: *How long is your menstrual cycle?*
Patient: *Three to four days.*

Many people think that the length of a cycle is how long you bleed for, but this is a common misconception. Your *cycle* is actually the number of days from the start of one period until the start of the next.

Education about periods is pretty mediocre at best. In fact, at my school it was so dire that I genuinely thought a period was the contents of an egg cracking and being released through the vagina, which often makes me laugh when I think of the irony that I now spend my life explaining periods to others. But rest assured, I've done my fair share of reading since then.

In this chapter I want to start with the absolute basics, so do bear with me if you're a period pro, although I hope there will be something to be gained for you geeks too.

If you fall into the 'I'm-in-need-of-period-101' group, you are not alone. A recent survey by ActionAid UK revealed that one in four women in the UK does not understand her periods, and that 20 per cent feel embarrassed to talk to their friends about them. If we can't talk about periods, we will never work out what is normal or abnormal. And this results in so many women suffering unnecessarily because they don't realise that there are things that can be done to help the problems they experience on a monthly basis.

What is a period?

A period is what happens when the lining of the uterus (the endometrium) falls away. Even though most of us are not trying to get pregnant the majority of the time, the entire reason for having a menstrual cycle is to prepare your uterus for a fertilised egg to implant. When this doesn't happen, your uterus chucks out the lining it had prepared. But in order to actually have a period there is a lot of work going on behind the scenes throughout the menstrual cycle.

'Day 1' is the first day of your period. If you have a text-book twenty-eight-day cycle, Day 28 is therefore the last day before your next period. We are, however, humans, of course, and not everyone goes by the book, with only about 15 per cent of women actually having a twenty-eight day cycle,[1] and anything between twenty-one and thirty-five days being considered a 'normal' cycle length.

The menstrual cycle: more than just a bit of bleeding

Let me take you through the different stages of your cycle.

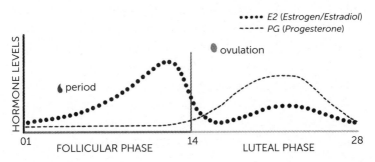

Follicular phase: fifty shades of period blood

It all starts on 'Day 1' – this is the first day of your period – and the bleeding usually lasts for three to eight days (on average five). Bleeding is classically heaviest on Day 2.

The blood during your period can come in a huge range of shades and hues. It won't look the same as the blood you see when you cut your finger, because it's not just plain blood. It's mixed with mucus and cells from the inside of the uterus and the reason there is blood in the first place is because the juicy lining that's built up over the month contains an intricate network of blood vessels that were meant to feed that elusive pregnancy it was planning on accommodating. The colour also depends on the time taken for the blood to come out. Just as an apple goes brown when it is cut and left exposed to the air, so blood starts to darken and, ultimately, go brown or almost black if it's left to hang around for long enough.

It's not uncommon for a period to start as spotting. This means light bleeding that's not really enough to need a pad. It can be pinkish, which is usually due to the lining starting to fall away, or various shades of brown, which means it's coming out very slowly or could even be old blood from your last period. Don't be overwhelmed by this; it's normal. New red bleeding tends to be thinner and often a bit watery because it's the freshest. It can get a bit thicker and more crimson in colour because it has had a bit of a wait before show itself. Then normally it becomes quite light and turns brown to black before it stops completely. A wide range of colours is completely normal and to be expected.

The blood that's being shed will clot in the uterus, so your body has to make anticoagulants – chemicals to break them down – in order to re-liquify the blood, so it can flow out. Many women tell me that 'pieces of liver are coming out'. Admittedly, clots may look pretty sinister, but it's not always something to worry about. If the amount of blood present exceeds the speed at which your body can make these anticoagulants you may experience clots, which can escape through your cervix, which softens slightly to allow the blood to escape. Clots tend to be small, usually no bigger than the size of a fifty-pence coin. However, larger clots, and lots of them, are a sign that there's heavy bleeding going on, so it's worth visiting your GP to check it's not causing anaemia, to consider treatment and whether there's an underlying reason, many of which are covered in Chapter 5.

While you've been busy concentrating on the outward manifestations of your period, you may not have realised that your brain has been busy making hormones: GnRH (gonadotrophin-releasing hormone), LH (luteinising hormone) and FSH (follicle-stimulating hormone). GnRH is produced first by the hypothalamus and then signals to the anterior pituitary to release LH and FSH, which then stimulate the ovary to prepare an egg for release (ovulation) and to produce oestrogen, which starts to rebuild the endometrium, in preparation for the hope of a pregnancy during this new cycle. Eventually, there is a massive surge in LH release, which triggers ovulation. LH is what you are trying to detect with the ovulation sticks that you can buy if you're trying to get pregnant and want to work out when you're ovulating. A patient once proudly told me that she usually ovulates about three times per month because her ovulation sticks told her so. You cannot ovulate more than once during a single menstrual cycle, although you can release more than one egg, which is how you get non-identical twins. This is one of the quirks of ovulation sticks; they tell you when you have had an LH surge, which can happen several times in one cycle, but they don't confirm you popped out an egg.

Luteal phase: eggs and shells

Eggs live in sacs called 'follicles' which undergo several months of maturation before they can get to the stage of being released. Ovulation marks the start of the luteal phase and is like a Hollywood audition; at the start of your cycle there may be ten eager, willing candidates, but as time goes on, only one is selected to go forward and become the 'dominant follicle', which grows and grows, forming a cyst which pops on about Day 12–16 of the cycle, throwing it on to the main stage in the hope of being fertilised. It's not unusual to get a bit of pain at this point. Ovulation itself is an inflammatory process and the ovary producing the 'star egg of the show' can get slightly enlarged which itself causes pain; then, when the cyst bursts, it leaks a little bit of fluid into your pelvis which can be uncomfortable. This ovulation pain (also called 'mittelschmerz', German for 'middle pain') can be sharp or like toothache, really low down near your hip bone on one side, but it usually lasts only twelve to twenty-four hours. Many women are quite anxious about this kind of pain and are horrified by the idea of a cyst bursting in their tummies. But it's a positive sign that their bodies are working the way they should, which reassures most people. There may also be a little bit of bleeding at this time; ovulation bleeding only happens in about 3 per cent of cycles,[2] but it's certainly nothing abnormal that you need to worry about. It happens due to a momentary drop in oestrogen.

After the egg is released, a shell of the original follicle, called the 'corpus luteum' is left behind in the ovary, which starts to release progesterone – the pro-pregnancy hormone. One of its main roles is to ensure the lining is fully preened and plumped up for the arrival of a fertilised egg. Progesterone levels are at their highest seven days after ovulation, and if fertilisation has not occurred, the corpus luteum eventually throws its hands up in the air and says, 'I can't do this any more. I'm bored of pumping out all this progesterone to no avail. I'm out of here!' It then slowly starts to degrade, and this causes a drop in both oestrogen and progesterone, which means the growth of the endometrium is no longer supported, so it begins to fall away. This is your period and the cycle starts again.

Variations in cycle length

It's normal for there to be some variation in the length of your menstrual cycle on a month-to-month basis.

A lot of mums of teenage girls contact me online, worried that there is something wrong with their daughters because they are only having periods every two or three months. But this is quite common when your periods start because the hormone cycles are still synchronising, and also coming up to the menopause when you have fewer eggs left, meaning you're less likely to ovulate as easily. Cycles are typically shortest and most regular in your twenties and thirties. Any variation in the length of the cycle at any age will be due to changes in the follicular phase because the length of the luteal phase is pretty standard being dictated by the lifespan of the corpus luteum.[3] (See Chapter 4 for other factors affecting cycle length besides age.)

Menstrual cups, tampons, pads . . . ?

There are an overwhelming number of 'menstrual-hygiene' products on the market; I'm not hugely keen on the term because I think it perpetuates the myth of periods being 'dirty'.

Menstrual cups, tampons, pads . . . I'm constantly asked which are 'the best', and, to be honest, from a health point of view there is no shining star – so I'd advise you to use whichever makes you feel most comfortable.

Menstrual cups

There may be a few furrowed brows at the mention of 'menstrual cups'. If you are wondering, they are small and egg-cup-shaped and made of a soft silicone, which you insert into your vagina, where they sit collecting blood as it comes out of the cervix. There's only one small study that has ever compared tampons and cups head to head and actually found greater satisfaction with cups compared to tampons, but it didn't find any difference in terms of infections[4] and there don't appear to be any clear health benefits. The main advantage is that they are probably better for the environment and will definitely save you money in the long run. But don't feel you have to use them. I don't recommend them for the squeamish, as you have to be quite cool about putting your fingers into your vagina to insert them (they don't come with an applicator like tampons), and it takes a bit of patience to learn how to remove them. After writing an Instagram post on menstrual cups I received a flurry of messages from women sharing the horror stories and proud moments of their first time. The most common initial problem seems to be difficulty removing it. Do not underestimate the strength of the vacuum that a menstrual cup can make with the cervix. However, you'll quickly learn how to break the vacuum and remove it like a pro.

I'm frequently asked if it's OK to use them with a contraceptive coil. Different manufacturers have different ideas on this, some saying it's OK, others saying it should be avoided. This is because theoretically you could dislodge your coil with the aforementioned vacuum effect – something that has, in fact, been confirmed by several women who have contacted me via social media saying they managed to suction out their coil: 'Anita, I've saved my coil, can you put it back in?' was one SOS message I recently received from a friend. But while I'm all for recycling, you can't reuse a coil, so I promptly replied, 'Sorry, darling, you need a fresh one!' If you do choose to use a cup with a coil, I would advise checking the strings at the end of your period. If you feel they are lower than normal, you can feel the rod of the coil or you can't feel any strings at all, I would use condoms until you've had it checked by a doctor to ensure it's still in the right place to give you full contraceptive protection.

Tampons

Just as menstrual cups may not be for everyone, the same goes for tampons. Some women just don't feel comfortable putting something inside themselves. Others find it too painful. This may be due to tight pelvic-floor muscles or not being relaxed enough or, in my experience, endometriosis, probably due to inflammation and scarring in the pelvis. One study suggested that tampon use is protective against endometriosis,[5] but I think this finding is skewed by the fact that a lot of patients with endometriosis don't use tampons because it's too uncomfortable to put them in or because their period is so heavy that a tampon isn't going to cut it.

Toxic-shock syndrome

Toxic-shock syndrome (TSS) is caused by bacteria and has nothing to do with any kind of chemical that is in the tampon itself. *Staphylococcus aureus* is a type of bacteria commonly found on the skin, and a particular form can produce a toxin called TSST-1. On entering the bloodstream, this can cause a massive inflammatory reaction, usually characterised by a really high fever, vomiting, skin rashes and aching muscles.

But, unhelpfully, it doesn't always lead to any symptoms 'down there' which would make it easier to identify the cause. It can be life-threatening and requires urgent medical attention. It's also incredibly rare, with only about forty cases per year in the UK, around half of which are thought to be related to tampon use (the other half are seen in children, men and older women, and are typically associated with skin burns and infections).

The ways that tampon use can potentially increase the risk of TSS include:

- collecting blood and increasing vaginal pH to create a breeding ground for bacteria
- causing tiny little micro-tears in the vaginal wall on insertion and removal, which allow bacteria to enter the bloodstream (it has been suggested that menstrual cups are safer in this regard, although I disagree; there has been a reported case of TSS with menstrual-cup use,[6] probably because it too can cause vaginal abrasions and potentially create the right bacterial breeding ground.

On balance, I don't think there's any reason for the social media-based frenzy related to tampons, or enough evidence for changing your practices, especially because TSS is so rare.

Pads

Let's not forget pads now. They might not be the sexy option these days, but they're still incredibly useful, especially for light days, and a godsend to the many women who don't like tampons or cups. To be clear, you don't need the scented ones, which some women find cause irritation to the delicate vulval tissue. Reusable pads, as well as periods pants, with an inbuilt absorbable pad, are also increasingly popular. These are better for the environment, and there's no difference between them and disposable pads from a health perspective.

||||||||||||||||||||||||||||||||||||||||

THINGS YOU'VE ALWAYS WANTED TO KNOW, BUT WERE TOO AFRAID TO ASK

Should I track my menstrual cycle?

I'm a massive fan of cycle tracking and usually recommend the Clue app (see Resources, page 242). It stops you being caught short without pads or tampons and can be really useful in helping you to recognise patterns in symptoms that you might get at particular times of the month. I breathe a sigh of relief when a patient gets her phone out to tell me all about her periods because it makes things so much easier to pinpoint; and if you haven't been doing it, we will often give you a menstrual-cycle tracking chart to fill in for the next few months.

I started tracking my period as a way of reassuring myself that the pain in my side every month was ovulation pain and not some dreadful case of appendicitis; all doctors are hypochondriacs to some extent. I did my medical-school elective on a tiny island in Fiji, where I had what I now realise was terrible ovulation pain, but at the time I was panicking and planning how I would get airlifted out to get my appendix removed because I didn't want to undergo surgery in our operating theatre, which was essentially a shed with a bright light. It was the worst twelve hours of my life! (And I've also seen the occasional woman arrive at A&E with the same fear.)

What is a fake period?

I've heard people referring to periods on the Pill as 'fake periods', which can cause a bit of anxiety. What they mean is that the bleeding is due to the hormones in the Pill, unlike a 'true period', in which the bleeding is caused by your body making the necessary hormones. When you stop taking your Pill it mimics the last few days in your cycle where the corpus luteum is dying away, so the levels of synthetic hormones from the Pill are dropping, which causes the lining to fall away.

I'm often asked: 'If it's a fake period, does that mean I could still be pregnant?' And the answer is, 'No'. If you have a bleed on the Pill when you have your week-long break, then you are not pregnant.

Are organic tampons better?

Many concerned women have contacted me asking if they're harming themselves by using conventional tampons, which, if you believe the hype, contain bleach plus cancer- and endometriosis-causing toxins. These claims are entirely unfounded, as very sophisticated lab techniques have failed to pick up any of these compounds in non-organic tampons.[7] Dioxins are a type of toxin that seem to get the most attention, but you actually ingest way more of these through your diet than you ever could through a humble tampon.[8] At present there is no scientific evidence to show organic tampons are better for health or *any less likely to be associated with TSS*. But they're definitely more expensive.

Some people have said they find organic tampons less irritating, and while there's no specific mechanism for why that might be the case, if you do find you're not satisfied with your current brand, you have nothing to lose by changing to an organic brand to see if it makes a difference. But my medical (and non-medical) opinion is: if it ain't broke, don't try to fix it.

Can I stop my period if I'm going on holiday?
Yes, and there are two ways to do so.

If you're on the combined oral contraceptive pill (COCP)
The COCP is the type you take for twenty-one days and then have a break for seven days, during which you would have your period. If you want to stop your period, it's OK to take up to three packs in a row without a break. You won't have a bleed because you maintain a constant hormone level, although some people will find they get some cramping and spotting, especially towards the end of the third pack.

If you're not on the COCP In this case, your GP can prescribe Norethisterone, a synthetic progestogen tablet that you take three times per day, starting about ten days before your period is due and continuing for the duration of your trip/the time for which you want to stop your period. Your period will usually start about two days after stopping the tablets. Again, they can cause cramping and spotting and your period might be heavier than normal.

There isn't a 'non-hormonal' way of stopping/delaying your period.

||||||||||||||||||||||||||||||||||||||||||||

THE GYNAE GEEK'S
KNOWLEDGE
BOMBS

I love a good ol' period chat. I always find that it's something everyone wants to talk about, but no one wants
to be the first to bring it up, whether in clinic or socially.
One of my biggest missions is to help start this conversation, so that you can understand what's normal and
when something might need medical attention. Here are
the five key points that I've covered in this chapter that I
find myself repeating over and over:

- A period is what happens when the lining of the uterus
  falls away, containing blood, mucus and old cells. It's
  not your body detoxing itself, it just means you didn't
  get pregnant.
- Your period blood can be like a rainbow – pinks, reds,
  browns, blacks; they're all normal.
- It's common to have irregular, often quite long cycles at
  the extremes of your menstrual life – as a teenager and
  before the menopause.
- Menstrual cups, tampons, pads – there isn't one
  outstanding product. Use what makes you feel
  comfortable.
- Toxic-shock syndrome is exceedingly rare, so again, use
  whichever product you prefer.

CHAPTER 4

Irregular and absent periods

I used to dread the time when my period arrived, but now I'm desperate to have one . . . what can I do?

Irregular periods are something I hear about frequently in clinic and get a lot of messages about online. Sometimes absent for months on end, they can cause a lot of stress, often because women worry they're going to struggle to get pregnant eventually. There's been a lot of media interest in polycystic ovarian syndrome (PCOS) lately, and while it's a common cause of a disrupted cycle, many people don't realise the impact that our hectic lifestyles can also have on periods. Most women tell me that they always had a regular cycle right from the word go, but that more recently they've gone completely haywire.

This is something that happened to me, and I had absolutely no idea of why. I'd thought my body was normal, so why had it started misbehaving? What I didn't appreciate (and was never taught in medical school) was that my body was warning me that my intense exercise regime, lack of sleep and through-the-roof stress levels were putting it under incredible strain and destroying any hope of a normal menstrual cycle. Let me explain how and why these things alter your period and, while I'm at it, I will also give you a good rundown of PCOS.

How irregular is irregular?

Many people believe that anything that is not a twenty-eight-day cycle is irregular, but if your period comes, for example, every twenty-six to thirty days, that's regular for you. As doctors, when we use the term 'irregular', we are talking about a cycle that has no rhyme or reason. This means you generally cannot predict when your period is going to come, and the variation in cycle length is usually more than ten days (i.e. If your shortest cycle is twenty-five days and the longest is sixty, the variation is thirty-five days). 'Amenorrhoea' is the term used when you don't have a period for at least three or six months (depending on your source). It is also very common and something that causes a great deal of anxiety.

'Lazy ovaries' are not 'a thing'

I've heard of people being told they are not having periods because of 'lazy ovaries', which is a bit unfair, as those poor little ovaries are trying their hardest to 'keep calm and carry on'. Your menstrual cycle is not just controlled by your ovaries; they rely on getting the appropriate signals from the brain – the hypothalamus and anterior pituitary gland being the two areas that make the hormones that communicate with the ovaries to stimulate oestrogen and progesterone production. Many things can interfere with this communication, changing your menstrual cycle as a result.

Causes of irregular or absent periods

I'm sure a number of the issues outlined below will resonate with a lot of you, and if they do, I suggest you hotfoot it to Part Five for a more thorough insight into these factors.

Note: it may sound obvious but the first thing you need to check for when you're not having a period is . . . pregnancy.

Hypothalamic amenorrhoea (HA)

Also called functional amenorrhoea, this is one of the most common topics I am contacted about via email and social media, usually by women who say things like; 'I haven't had a period for over a year and I just can't understand why. I exercise five times a week and I'm on a really healthy diet.' Although I have no statistics to back this up, I would estimate that it is more common in young, fit women heavily invested in a healthy lifestyle. Unfortunately, the current fashion for an athletic physique, combined with the 'more-is-more' attitude of society and our hectic lifestyles leave little room for the simple things in life – like hormone production. That is why women get HA; and I can usually tell this straight away from the Instagram profiles of the many women who message me about this problem – their bodies have quite simply run out of steam.

While we may not be very good at consciously prioritising the essentials, our bodies do this automatically as a way of helping us to survive. As over-the-top as it sounds, your body would prefer to keep your heart beating, rather than give you a period, so your brain shuts off production of the hormones that stimulate your ovaries, which stops ovulation. And since the entire purpose of your menstrual cycle is for you to get pregnant, Mother Nature is particularly clever, recognising that a stressed-out woman does not need the added stress of having a baby. From an evolutionary point of view, this is a survival tactic for both mother and baby.

The main triggers for hypothalamic amenorrhoea that I see on a recurrent basis are stress, diet and overexercising – or, usually, a combination of all three.

Stress

You've probably heard of cortisol, the stress hormone. It influences production of female hormones by telling your brain that you're under stress (even if you don't realise it) and to halt ovulation until you've overcome it. Unfortunately, we are so used to living our lives in 'turbo-power mode' that we've forgotten what it's really like to press the pause button, or even that it exists. I frequently meet real-life superwomen. They typically have several children, a zoo-worth of animals and a husband who isn't very domesticated. And often an irregular cycle. Recently, I called one of these superwomen into my room and apologised that the clinic was running late. She said, 'Oh, don't worry; it's been lovely to sit and read a magazine and have some time to myself . . . ' So before she'd even sat down I was pretty certain of what the problem was, although it can be a tricky one to solve because so many women have lost sight of how important it is to take that critical time for themselves.

Dietary factors

If you're not eating enough to be able to provide the energy requirements of your own body, you're not going to be able to sustain a healthy pregnancy. So here again, your brain shuts the system down, saving the energy and nutrients that would otherwise be used on ovulation. Fat tissue is one of the sites of oestrogen production, so women with very low body fat may not produce enough oestrogen, which is made from a specific type of fat called cholesterol. Fat tissue is also able to send signals to the brain to tell it whether there is enough of the stuff to maintain a pregnancy. Female hormones are made of fats, so if your diet is devoid of good, healthy fats, your body doesn't have the right ingredients to make the goods.

I recently had a difficult conversation with a patient who had become a vegan right around the time that her periods stopped, but she was convinced that couldn't be the reason why, because to her, veganism was the healthiest diet out there. However, any extreme change in diet can lead to nutrient deficiency (see Chapter 14).

Overexercising

Adrenaline is the 'fight-or-flight' hormone that is going to save you from that wild bear. Nowadays, there are very few bears or other life-threatening mammals running around, but your body doesn't know the difference between thrashing it out on the treadmill or running from said bear. Your body senses this exertion as a stress and says to your ovaries, 'Hold your horses! This woman is in danger – do not ovulate.' It's common for long-distance runners to lose their periods, but it's not just running that can be a problem. Any intensive exercise can have the same effect. Many women that I see are training like athletes, then running off to their full-time jobs, families and social commitments and it can be too much for their bodies to cope with. They can also be putting themselves in a calorie deficit if they're not eating enough, which takes us back to dietary factors. All of this – and how to address it – is discussed further in Chapter 15 (see pages 212–226).

Post-Pill amenorrhoea

After stopping the contraceptive Pill you will have your usual bleed, assuming you stopped at the end of the pack. But when is your next period going to come? That's the million-dollar question. Some people will go back to having a regular cycle pretty much straight away. Others sit and wait . . . and wait . . . and wait some more. And in my experience, this is much more common than the textbooks say. But if the Pill is out of your system after a day or so, why does this happen? There is no single answer. It's likely to be a combination of three factors:

The Pill essentially takes over your natural hormones, so it can take some time for them to get back into sync to the point where they can resume 'business as usual'.

The triggers for hypothalamic amenorrhoea (see page 41), which I find to be very common.

The possibility of an underlying problem such as PCOS, which has been masked by the Pill.

Premature menopause

Also referred to as premature ovarian failure/insufficiency (POF/POI), premature menopause is actually a misnomer. You run out of eggs when you go through the menopause, whereas with POF/POI your ovaries stop responding, despite still having eggs on the shelf. I can't even count the number of times I've had women come and cry in my clinic room, convinced this is happening to them when their period has gone AWOL. It takes a very simple blood test to confirm or refute the diagnosis (oestrogen levels will be low and FSH will be through the roof) and, thankfully, it's pretty uncommon, affecting about 1 in 100 women before the age of forty, and 5 in 100 before forty-five (the average age in the UK for menopause being about fifty-one years). It tends to run in families, so asking your mum when she went through the menopause is helpful.

Hormonal diseases

PCOS is the most common hormonal disorder that can affect your periods and is discussed at length below. Diseases associated with hormones that seem unrelated to your ovaries can also have a dramatic impact due to the interconnection of the hormonal system as a whole. Thyroid disease (high or low levels) is particularly common in women, and changes in thyroid hormones have both a direct and indirect effect on female hormone levels, which can change the timing of your periods and also how heavy they are (see page 60). A thyroid blood test can be done by your GP, and this can reveal thyroid problems in many women. Type 1 diabetes (where your body is unable to make insulin) and type 2 diabetes (where your body becomes less responsive to insulin) are both associated with irregular cycles due to the interaction of insulin and female hormone production.[9,10] Type 2 diabetes can also be associated with PCOS, as described below. There are, of course, other hormonal diseases which, although less common, will be checked with blood tests.

Polycystic ovarian syndrome (PCOS)

This is the most common hormonal disorder seen in women, with some studies suggesting that up to 1 in 5 of us is affected. It is diagnosed based on the presence of two out of the following three characteristics known as the Rotterdam Criteria:

o Irregular or absent periods
o Signs of excess male hormones including excess body/facial hair or acne or high levels on a blood test
o Polycystic ovaries seen on an ultrasound scan

PCOS does not typically cause pain. Polycystic ovaries are often seen on scans to investigate lower abdominal pain, but are not the cause of this pain.

What causes PCOS?

PCOS is a syndrome (i.e. a collection of symptoms), so it's not the same cause in everyone. It is a complex mash-up of your in-built genetics, epigenetics (which is how genes are turned on and off) combined with environmental aspects of how we live our lives now.

One of the key features of PCOS is insulin-resistance, which is found in about 70 per cent of sufferers. This is when your body is able to make plenty of insulin (one of the key hormones responsible for keeping your blood sugar under control), but your tissues are less sensitive to it, and therefore you have to ramp up production to maintain the same response. The problem is that insulin forces your ovaries to convert oestrogen to the male hormone testosterone, which stops ovulation (goodbye regular periods) and gives you all the fun hormonal side effects (hello acne, excess hair, mood swings . . .). Blood tests and ultrasound scans are carried out to confirm it and rule out other causes of the symptoms.

So what causes PCOS in those who are not insulin resistant? The adrenal glands. As well as making cortisol, and the fight-or-flight hormones adrenaline and noradrenaline, they also make testosterone and its precursors, resulting in the same effect on your ovaries.

Management of PCOS
A lot of women are understandably disappointed to hear that there is no cure for PCOS. But there are plenty of ways to treat the symptoms, both through lifestyle changes and prescribed medication:

Lifestyle intervention
Every guideline I've ever come across for PCOS cites 'lifestyle intervention' as the first-line treatment, although doctors have not always been famed for giving the best lifestyle advice. Thankfully, times are changing and there is a new wave of doctors coming on to the scene, led by the likes of

my friends Dr Rupy Aujla, Dr Hazel Wallace and Dr Rangan Chatterjee (see Resources, page 242), all of whom dish out great lifestyle tips via their social-media platforms and chart-topping podcasts, so check them out.

Several years ago, a hugely overweight twenty-two-year-old came to clinic for advice about PCOS as she was planning on getting pregnant in the next few years. I spent about fifteen minutes talking to her all about lifestyle interventions that she could undertake. I gave her so many in-depth, practical tips and tricks that she could use to improve her PCOS and, in turn, her long-term health in general, which is so important for anyone planning a pregnancy, with or without PCOS. My heart sank though when she looked at me and said, 'But can't you just prescribe me a tablet to sort it all out?' Granted, these interventions are not easy, requiring some hard work and diligence at times, but you will reap the benefits in the long term because they can reduce the risk of the complications of PCOS, including type 2 diabetes and heart and vascular diseases, which are some of the major causes of death and chronic-health issues in the Western world.

Here is a summary of the advice that I give to my patients (see Part Five, pages 185–238, for more details).

○ **Weight loss** Many patients are surprised when I tell them I'm not going to ask them to lose weight. Weight loss *is* one of the most effective ways to help the symptoms of PCOS (reducing fat reduces insulin resistance, which is the main driver of the condition), making your cycles more regular, increasing the chance of a healthy pregnancy, improving acne and reducing the risk of diabetes and heart disease in the future.[11] *However*, being told to lose weight is psychologically tough and, I believe, makes the whole disease much more traumatic to deal with. I prefer instead to focus on improving diet and exercise which, if done correctly, will result in both improved symptoms and weight loss without this being a depressing focal point.

- **Diet** There are a lot of people pushing extreme PCOS diets online, particularly focused around low-carb/ketogenic (high-fat, low-carb) diets, which I don't subscribe to at all. The rationale behind them is sound, and data supports short-term effectiveness.[12] But we don't know for sure if these diets have a direct impact in the long term, and they're hard to stick to, so I don't recommend them unless a patient is insistent on trying. I also don't want to promote faddy eating in young, impressionable women, who are already at a higher risk of eating disorders.[13] Low-carb diets also run the risk of resulting in a low-fibre intake, which is associated with a higher risk of PCOS.[14]

  To get enough fibre, you need to eat carbs. Carbs are not the devil, but the devil is in the detail. You need to eat good-quality, high-fibre carbs such as oats, brown rice and fruits and veggies that are also packed with other precious nutrients that your body needs for all the complex chemical processes such as ovulation. Good-quality fats (see pages 202–3) are also essential because female hormones are made from cholesterol that is a fat. If you don't have the building blocks, you can't make the goods. The Mediterranean diet really is the one that has it all (see page 207 for more on that).

- **Exercise** Probably one of the questions I am most frequently asked online is: 'What's the best exercise for PCOS?' And my honest answer is: the one you're going to stick with – because dealing with PCOS is about being consistent. And exercise doesn't have to happen in a gym either; so for many people, something as simple as going for a walk at lunchtime or getting off the bus a few stops early may be exactly what they need and what fits with their schedule. If you want to get geeky about it, one of the main aims of exercise for PCOS is to slightly alter body composition to increase lean muscle and decrease fat tissue (see Chapter 15). Muscle is much more sensitive to insulin compared to fat, and also needs more energy, so improves your metabolism.

○ **Relaxation** Life is stressful. Stress increases cortisol, which increases insulin resistance and testosterone levels. If you can remove the driver, you can break the cycle. Realistically, we can't take all the stress out of our lives – and nor should we, as a certain amount of stress is good for us – but we have to look for ways to manage it. Depression and anxiety levels are also known to be higher in women with PCOS,[15] so self-care is very important. Exercise is a great way of addressing self-care and helping you to relax.

○ **Sleep** Lack of sleep makes you more insulin resistant, as well as causing cravings for sweet, fatty, high-calorie, low-nutrient foods and caffeine, all of which spike cortisol. And the vicious PCOS cycle continues to turn. I find that exercise helps me sleep better, so as you can see, all the things in this section go hand in hand.

Medication

This isn't an exhaustive list, but these are the three types of medication that I get asked about the most:

○ **The Pill** The combined oral contraceptive Pill (COCP) will not 'balance your hormones'. While it is entirely acceptable to use the Pill to ensure you have a regular monthly bleed, or as contraception, it will not treat the underlying cause of your irregular cycle. Once you decide to stop taking the Pill your periods will likely still be irregular, unless you've made some serious lifestyle changes. I see a lot of patients in clinic who are very disappointed to hear this as they're under the impression that by using the Pill, their PCOS is cured; it isn't. The Pill just forces the body to bleed on the week off.

Many women are not keen on taking the Pill, but it is advised to have at least four periods per year to reduce the risk of the uterine lining becoming too thick and irregular which can, in the long run, increase the risk of endometrial cancer. The other advantage of the Pill is that it helps your body to make something called 'sex hormone-binding globulin', which mops up excess testosterone, so helping with acne and excess hair.

○ **Metformin** This is a diabetes medication that reduces insulin resistance. A lot of women tell me they hate it though because it can cause awful stomach cramps and diarrhoea. While metformin can be effective for improving ovulation, body weight and composition, it works best when used in conjunction with lifestyle modification.[16]

○ **Inositol** This is a dietary supplement that can be bought over the counter. Of all the many supplements that have been proposed for use in PCOS this one seems to get the most coverage online and, thankfully, has the biggest evidence base, relatively speaking. I've seen a really positive effect from inositol in quite a few women; however, although lab studies suggest it may reduce insulin resistance, and there has been a handful of small human studies to show it can improve menstrual-cycle regularity, reduce testosterone and even increase the chance of pregnancy,[17] there haven't yet been any big trials to prove exactly how effective it is, the best type to use or the optimum dose, so it's not something that's routinely recommended by many gynaecologists just yet.

||||||||||||||||||||||||||||||||||||||||||

THINGS YOU'VE ALWAYS WANTED TO KNOW, BUT WERE TOO AFRAID TO ASK

When should irregular periods be investigated?

There is no hard-and-fast rule. A sensible approach would be to see your GP if you are having periods less often than every three months, or if you've recently started having an irregular cycle. A lot of patients say they've always had an irregular cycle, but this should still be investigated as there may be a correctable cause.

I frequently receive messages from concerned mothers, such as: 'My fifteen-year-old daughter has had irregular periods ever since they started three years ago and her GP won't do anything about it.' While it's bound to be worrying, remember that it can be normal for teenagers to have irregular periods and may take about five years from when they start to settle down into a more regular cycle.[18] So it's not always wrong to leave things alone to see if they sort themselves out, but it very much depends on what else is going on and what other symptoms she may be having, so do discuss this with your GP if you are worried.

Are there any health risks associated with hypothalamic amenorrhoea?

First and foremost, the thing that most women are worried about is fertility. If you're not ovulating, you can't get pregnant.

So if you want to have a baby in the near future, you need to speak to your doctor as soon as possible.

One of the biggest risks with HA, however – and many women are not aware of this – is the risk of brittle bones and heart disease that can arise due to a lack of oestrogen, which I would suggest is just as important as your fertility. I'm really passionate about ensuring this message filters through. We often tend to focus on short-term, tangible outcomes, forgetting the things we can't see. 'I'd rather look shredded now and deal with my bones when I get older,' one patient told me. But that's the problem. You can't deal with your bones later. Peak bone strength in females occurs around the age of thirty, and if you're not building it in those crucial teens and twenties you can't catch up later. Build it now, for benefits down the line.

Does PCOS increase the risk of ovarian cancer?

This is the thing that everyone worries about. PCOS itself does not increase your risk of getting ovarian cancer,[19] but obesity and diabetes, both of which are associated with PCOS, may do so. It's important, therefore, to try and implement some of the lifestyle changes discussed on page 54.

PCOS does increase the risk of endometrial cancer (cancer of the lining of the uterus),[20] the greatest risk being to women who are less physically active, regardless of obesity or diabetes.[21] So anything you can do to increase the amount of movement you do may reduce your risk, irrespective of whether you actually lose weight,[22] which is another reason why I prefer to steer away from concentrating on weight loss as a specific goal.

I had a scan that shows I have polycystic ovaries – what are the implications of this?

'Polycystic' means having lots of cysts. With regards to your ovaries, this means you have loads of follicles that are trying to mature and break free. Up to 25 per cent of women have ovaries with a polycystic appearance,[23] and it's particularly common in younger girls who have started their periods in the last few years because their ovaries are literally bursting with eggs wanting to get out. However, it doesn't automatically mean you have polycystic ovarian syndrome (PCOS), if you don't have any of the other classic symptoms (see page 45).

||||||||||||||||||||||||||||||||||||||||

THE GYNAE GEEK'S KNOWLEDGE BOMBS

Irregular or absent periods cause so much anxiety, so I hope this chapter will have put your mind at ease, giving you a few areas of your life to re-evaluate if this is a particular problem for you. The most important takeaways here are:

- Lazy ovaries do not exist. If you stop having periods it's because your ovaries aren't receiving the right messages from the brain, or other hormones are influencing their activity.
- Premature menopause is very rare and unlikely to be the cause of irregular or absent periods, but it is very easy to check for with a simple blood test.
- Your body is very clever and is able to stop your periods if you are stressed, overexercising or not eating well, as a survival tactic to conserve energy for things that are more important than making hormones.
- The contraceptive Pill will not cure PCOS. It will merely cause you to have a period every month, but when you stop the Pill, if you haven't made any lifestyle changes, your body will resume the same cycle as before you started it.
- Lifestyle changes including diet, exercise and stress management can have a massive positive impact on PCOS. They also reduce your risk of complications such as diabetes, heart disease and female cancers.

CHAPTER 5

Heavy periods and other period-related frustrations

'I hate leaving the house on the first few days of my period because I'm so scared of leaking through my clothes.'

If you skipped the introduction to this book you need to go right back there and read the story on pages xi–xiii, which illustrates how horrendous periods can be and the dramatic impact they can have on women's lives.

I'm sure you know someone who has terrible periods, but they may not talk to you about it, and, as a result, many of us don't know what other people's periods are like, or even whether our own are 'normal'. As a result, many women feel ashamed, and so they suffer in silence, not leaving the house for the first few days due to pain or needing to change their pads constantly, or through fear of leaking.

There are a lot of things that can be done to improve the situation, but your doctor has to actually know that you are having problems, so don't be afraid to go and talk to them about it. As doctors, we're not fazed by things you wouldn't dare tell anyone else, nor do we expect you to use any complex medical lingo. I can usually tell when a patient is shy and embarrassed, and try and use all the awkward words in my first few questions, just to prove to them that it really is safe to say whatever they want to.

My advice is to keep it simple by giving a basic explanation of what's going on in language that you feel comfortable using and your doctor will use their expertise to ask you for more info.

Heavy periods

One in five women will experience heavy periods, also known as menorrhagia – literally, raging periods. Let's look at what this means.

How heavy is heavy?

The textbooks state that anything over 80ml blood loss is classified as heavy. But what does that even mean? No one sits over a jug and measures it, and it's incredibly difficult to quantify the amount on a sanitary pad or tampon. A more helpful way of classifying a heavy period would be any of the following:

- Changing pads/tampons at least every hour for several hours in a row
- Needing to use a pad and a tampon at the same time
- Bleeding for longer than seven days
- Any excessive menstrual blood loss which interferes with the woman's physical, emotional, social and material quality of life, and which can occur alone or in combination with other symptoms

This last guideline come from the UK's National Institute of Health and Clinical Excellence (NICE) and, to me, is the most important – because everyone is different, and it doesn't matter what's acceptable to someone else, it's what's acceptable to you.

Feeling tired and having no energy during your period is very common (whether they are heavy or not). Many people worry it's from the blood loss. But if you compare it to the amount you give during a blood-donation session (470ml over about ten minutes) it's not actually that much, and it's been shown that only about 30–50 per cent of the fluid that is lost during a period is actually straight-up blood, the remainder being fluid that leaks out from the uterine lining.[24] So what's making you so tired? Most likely, it's the low oestrogen levels, so the tiredness should go when your period finishes. But if you feel it lasts longer, you should see your GP to check for anaemia (low haemoglobin levels) and other causes of tiredness. About two thirds of women with heavy periods are anaemic as a result.[25]

Causes of heavy periods

About 50 per cent of cases have no identifiable cause, which is called 'dysfunctional uterine bleeding'. This can only be diagnosed once other identifiable causes described below have been considered and eliminated.

Fibroids

These are benign (non-cancerous) overgrowths of the muscle of the wall of the uterus. About 10 per cent of women with heavy periods are known to have fibroids,[25] but not all of them experience heavy periods or any trouble at all. They can be tiny, or, in some cases, so huge you can look at least six months pregnant. One panic-stricken nineteen-year-old came to clinic having never had sex before, but all her family were convinced she was pregnant because of what turned out to be a huge fibroid that was the size of a football. Size isn't a predictor of the kind of symptoms experienced though, and this girl didn't have heavy periods at all. It's more about location: some grow outwards, away from the cavity, some grow just in the wall itself and some grow inwards, pushing into the cavity. It's the latter that tend to cause heavy bleeding because they increase the surface area of the uterus, so you've got more lining to shed.

You can also have more than one fibroid at a time. Another patient with a very long history of heavy periods lay on my couch sobbing as I examined her because she was sure she had cancer. I pressed gently on her abdomen and her uterus felt like a bag of oranges. 'You have a lot of fibroids,' I told her. 'How do you know?' she sobbed. 'I can feel them,' I explained. 'You can too if you want,' and I placed her hands on to her stomach. Sure enough, the fibroids were subsequently seen on a scan, and I'm pleased to say she didn't have cancer.

PCOS
Irregular, infrequent periods are classic features of PCOS. But they can also be heavier as a result because your lining has had longer to thicken up, so there's more to come away.

Bleeding disorders
Your body makes natural blood-clotting agents that are involved in limiting the amount of blood that you lose during a period. If these are deficient, you can get really heavy periods. This tends to present itself from a young age and I've looked after some girls who were diagnosed following periods so heavy they needed to be admitted for blood transfusions. It can be diagnosed using special blood tests. Many bleeding disorders are hereditary, such as von Willebrand disease, so you may already be aware of a family history.

Being overweight

Fat tissue is a major source of oestrogen which, as you by now know, acts to build up the uterine lining to make it nice and cosy for that fertilised egg that your body so desperately wants you to implant there. Higher oestrogen levels will lead to a thicker uterine lining, which results in a heavier period, quite simply because there is more to come away. Unfortunately, this is something I see quite commonly and it's often difficult to convince patients that their body weight can have an impact on their periods. I remember one lady who looked seriously unimpressed when I suggested she changed her eating habits and started some exercise. As she walked out of my room, I remember feeling I had failed, and thought to myself, At least I tried . . . A few months later, I bumped into her in the hospital corridor and she had lost weight, felt generally amazing as a result and was having lighter periods – all without medication. She thanked me and said, 'Doctor, the proof really is in the pudding!'

Thyroid problems

Usually an underactive thyroid, which is also associated with fatigue, hair loss, muscle weakness, cold intolerance and . . . heavy periods! This is because your thyroid hormones play a role in regulating female hormone production, as well as the clotting factors that are needed to stem the flow. Women are more likely to have thyroid problems than men, and thankfully, this one is usually simple to correct with medication.

Endometriosis

This is where tissue that is similar to the uterine lining is found outside of the womb. It tends to cause very painful periods, and they are likely to be heavier than in women without endometriosis, but it's not thought to be as a result of the disease itself, which I'll explain more about later (see pages 63–4).

Copper coil

You probably weren't expecting this one! The copper coil is all the rage these days, and while it is very effective as a contraceptive (more on that in Chapter 7), it does usually cause heavier periods. In fact, this is one of the most common reasons for it to be removed ahead of its 'best-before' date. Yet many women don't seem to be told this before having it put in and, as a good friend told me, 'My period went from that annoying light rain that ruins your hair to a tropical downpour!' The hormone coil (Mirena is the most common brand name; Jaydess, Kyleena are both newer versions), on the other hand, will generally make your periods much lighter, which is why many women prefer it.

OK, I'm convinced my period is classified as heavy. Now what?

Blood tests will be done to look for anaemia and other causes of heavy bleeding such as thyroid disease. In order to look for causes such as fibroids you will be offered either an ultrasound scan or a hysteroscopy. The ultrasound scan is ideally done internally, 'using that stick that looks like it came from Ann Summers', as a patient's mother once said in an attempt at reassuring her daughter, whose expression quickly changed from scared to highly embarrassed. A hysteroscopy uses a tiny telescope that is inserted through the cervix to look directly inside the uterus. It can be done either in clinic or under general anaesthetic. During this procedure we can often take tissue samples, remove polyps and even certain types of fibroids at the same time.

Period pain

Period pain, or 'dysmenorrhoea' in medical speak, affects up to 90 per cent of menstruating women.[26] It's most common to get it in the first few days of your period, or even the day before. It's down to prostaglandins, which are chemicals released by tissues that can cause very small contractions of the uterine muscle which help to shimmy the period blood down and out. Pain usually occurs in your lower abdomen, but it's not uncommon to also get it in your back, buttocks and thighs, due to the connection of the nerves that supply the pelvic area. A lot of women say that they don't want to take painkillers in case they mask something more serious, but this would be hard to do with over-the-counter tablets. And there are no awards for struggling through, so don't feel afraid to try something if you need to.

How can period pain be treated?

There are many ways to treat period pain, but let's start with tablets.

Painkillers

Paracetamol is the most commonly bought over-the-counter painkiller in the UK, and in spite of the fact you don't need a prescription, it can be incredibly effective. Studies have shown, however, that ibuprofen is better than paracetamol for period pain.[27] Both work by blocking the activity of the pain-causing prostaglandins, but via different pathways, so you can actually take them safely together – a suggestion which horrifies a lot of people. If you find you frequently need something more than these, that should prompt a trip to your GP to discuss other options.

Hormonal treatments

The combined oral contraceptive Pill has long been used to treat period pain. It reduces prostaglandins production, and less prostaglandin = less pain. The hormonal coil is another popular hormonal treatment, and while a lot of women are a bit scared to try it, a phenomenal number come skipping back a few months later reporting success.

Exercise

The idea of sliding into Lycra while on your period may fill many of you with dread, but exercise is actually a great strategy for tackling period pain.[28] It doesn't have to be a heavy session in the gym, just something simple like a good walk. (See Chapter 15 for more on this.)

Heat

A hot-water bottle can be a very simple way of easing period pain. Every now and then I'll see a patient who has been slightly overdoing it with the heat though, and I can tell because she'll have a characteristic skin discolouration that looks like a lace veil on her stomach. It occurs as a result of excess heat exposure and is called *erythema ab igne*, if you want the fancy Latin name. It usually sets off alarm bells and is an indication of a woman in pretty severe pain. In many cases there may be an underlying cause for this pain, and often this is endometriosis (see box opposite).

Lack of periods – when you're running a boob-milk factory

One thing a lot of women seem to love is the fact that breast-feeding stops their periods. And understandably so, because when you've got 500 other things to think about, as well as

ENDO-WHAT NOW?

Endometriosis is the growth of endometrial-like tissue (lining of the uterus) outside the uterus, commonly on the ovaries, bowel, bladder and even on the liver and lungs in rare cases. No one really knows how this happens. One theory is that period blood tracks backwards out of the tubes, and then an altered immune response enables it to grow. Regardless, however, it behaves like it would inside the uterus, growing, thickening and shedding like a period – except that it has nowhere to go. This causes excruciating period pain and also scar tissue, making the normally mobile internal organs of your pelvis stick together. Depending on exactly where the scar tissue is, it can cause pain during sex, when going to the toilet for either a number one or two and general chronic pain that goes on throughout the month.

Endometriosis isn't seen well on scans and needs to be diagnosed via keyhole surgery (a laparoscopy) at which point deposits of endometriosis can be removed and scar tissue broken down. It must be performed by a specialist endometriosis surgeon because it can be very tricky work. I've stood in theatre for up to five or six back-breaking hours assisting in such operations, but on reflection I always realise the ache in my back is nothing compared to the pain these women endure. I often see women who tell me they can't go to work or even look after their children due to the pain. Periods can be painful, but they shouldn't be so bad that your life stops for days on end every month. It's a sign you need to go and have a chat with your doctor.

Endometriosis and fertility

Fertility is one of the most common concerns upon receiving a diagnosis of endometriosis. There is a higher chance that you will find it difficult to get pregnant, but the two don't necessarily go hand in hand, and I've seen lots of women with really dreadful endometriosis who have got pregnant really easily. I also see a lot of patients who are diagnosed while being investigated for infertility. And the really upsetting thing here is that the vast majority report a long-standing history of the common endometriosis symptoms, and most say they just thought it was normal, or something they just had to tolerate as part of being a woman. This is one of the 101 reasons why we need to be more open about periods, and why you shouldn't feel afraid to go and talk to your GP if you're concerned. No one should ever feel that heavy, painful periods, pain during sex or when passing urine is something they just have to deal with. These symptoms don't automatically mean that you have endometriosis, but it's a diagnosis that is worth considering and they may require further investigation.

running around a little one, a period is the last thing you need to deal with. And that's why Mother Nature made it that way. Quite simply, it's a survival tactic. Breastfeeding prevents the brain from releasing the hormones that activate your ovaries – and hence your menstrual cycle – to stop you from getting pregnant, which would ultimately stop you from producing milk for the baby you're currently feeding.

It's difficult to predict when your periods will start again based on how much you're feeding. For some people it happens when they're still feeding a couple of times a day, and for others it's when they've stopped completely. I've seen a lot of people who have got pregnant while breastfeeding though, so do remember that the absence of your periods at this time is not a failsafe contraceptive.

PMS

For many women, these three letters, which stand for premenstrual syndrome, are more than just a bad mood and an ice-cream tub. Hormone fluctuations affect mood throughout the menstrual cycle. Low oestrogen levels in particular are known to decrease release of serotonin, the happy hormone, which may explain why you may experience low mood before your periods.[29]

In about 5 per cent of women PMS is much more extreme – a condition called premenstrual dysphoric disorder (PMDD).[30] On several occasions I've seen women who have asked to have their ovaries removed because their lives are turned upside down by hormones every month. Treatment may include the use of the Pill or antidepressants, but the best responses I have seen have been with cognitive behavioural therapy (CBT) and mindfulness.

Physical symptoms can also manifest in the lead-up to your period. There's nothing like a bit of PMS-induced bloating to make you freak out that you're actually pregnant, rather than about to have a period. And from what Instagram tells me these days, we've all been there, as there are loads of girls posting photos of their #periodbloat. It's refreshing to see women talking about this common problem, which is caused by water retention from the hormone progesterone. It's also the reason you can get breast swelling and tenderness. Sleep can also be affected and some people get terrible headaches or migraines.

PMS and PMDD are real conditions, and not something you're making up in your head as many women are led to think. No one really understands why some people get PMS or PMDD, although the latter is more common in women with a history of mental-health disorders.[30] There is certainly a role here for stress management, diet and exercise, however, and these will be covered later, in Part Five.

‖‖‖‖‖‖‖‖‖‖‖‖‖‖‖‖‖‖‖‖‖‖‖‖‖‖‖‖‖‖‖‖‖‖

THINGS YOU'VE ALWAYS WANTED TO KNOW, BUT WERE TOO AFRAID TO ASK

None of this applies to me. My period is super light. Is that abnormal?

If you've always had light periods, you're lucky! If they've recently become lighter, there may be an underlying reason that could require investigation. These include thyroid problems, being super stressed or having lost a lot of weight. I'm also seeing a lot of girls getting really light periods after extreme changes in diet, such as becoming vegan. I'll cover some of these things in Part Five. But if you're concerned, do see your GP.

Are heavy periods a sign of cancer? Or bleeding in between periods?

This is the thing that everyone is afraid of, but the answer is: infrequently. The risk of cancer with heavy periods is 0.1 per cent (1 in 1000),[31] which is why I didn't even list it above. I once called a thirty-year-old lady into my room in clinic, and as she sat down, she began crying uncontrollably. Never a good start to a consultation. Several minutes and half a box of cheap NHS tissues later, I learned that she had spent the previous six weeks unable to eat, sleep or care for her children because she was so convinced that she had cancer due to bleeding between her periods. I'm pleased to say that she didn't (the numbers are 0.5 per cent – 5 in 1,000 having cancer with this type of bleeding),[31] but don't be afraid to let your doctor know your concerns from the start, so that they can help and reassure you.

Can supplements help my painful periods?

There are a baffling number of supplements touted as 'the cure for period pain'. Unfortunately, there isn't currently a great deal of strong evidence for many of them[32] and, with magnesium, zinc, vitamins D and E, along with a whole host of others suggested to help in various studies at various doses, where do you even start? Personally, I think it's better (and more enjoyable) to try and get these nutrients into your body as part of a healthy diet (see Chapter 14 for more on this).

Do I need a hysterectomy if I have endometriosis?

The American actress Lena Dunham wrote an essay for *Vogue* about the hysterectomy that she had at the tender age of thirty-one after a long and very public battle with endometriosis. I'm sure it wasn't an easy decision for her to make, but I must stress this is not a routine treatment for endometriosis and is only reserved for a minority of cases where all other treatments, both medical and less drastic surgery, have failed.

It's almost impossible to remove all the deposits outside of the uterus, so there is a high chance of getting a recurrence of pain, especially if the ovaries are left behind to prevent premature menopause, although this can even happen when the ovaries are removed. Therefore, it's preferred to try other types of treatment first.

Is stress making my periods more painful?

It's very possible. Studies have shown stress can cause more painful periods and can even affect your cycle the following month as well. This is due to the interaction with the stress hormone cortisol and your female hormones, as well as the effect cortisol has on production of prostaglandins, the chemical responsible for period pain. I also see this with both my patients and myself, with house moves/renovations and marital problems being the most common factors cited (for me, it's night shifts; arguably, the lesser of the evils!).

Period sex – yay or nay?

Now that I've hopefully got you comfortable with at least thinking about, and maybe even talking about periods, I'm going to really go for it and finish off by talking about period sex – it's like Marmite: you either love it or hate it – and it can make a mess.

A lot of women say they feel most aroused during their period. From an evolutionary point of view, we are pro-grammed to want to have sex the most around ovulation to increase the chance of pregnancy, and this is the case because hormone levels are at their highest. But during your period, your hormones levels are at their lowest. So it doesn't quite make sense to have a high libido at this time. One theory relates to the fact that the pelvis may be engorged with blood, which can stimulate pelvic nerves leading to arousal. While it hasn't been proven, it's probably the only plausible mechanism I've heard so far.

It's worth noting that you can still get pregnant if you have sex during your period, particularly if you're someone who has a very short cycle, meaning you will ovulate very close to your period, so you should still use contraception. There is also a slightly higher risk of getting an STI during your period, due to changes in the immune system of the cervix, so a condom wouldn't go amiss if you aren't using any other contraception and/or haven't been screened for STIs (see Chapters 6 and 7 for more on this).

|||||||||||||||||||||||||||||||||||||||||||

THE GYNAE GEEK'S KNOWLEDGE BOMBS

We need to talk more about periods. It's the only way to understand what's normal and what's not. And a lack of this understanding is one of the reasons I see so many women who have suffered in silence for too long, thinking their symptoms were 'normal' or something they needed to put up with. I hope this chapter has given you some pointers about whether your period needs any attention. Please remember the following:

○ One in five women suffers from heavy periods. Far too many women delay visiting a doctor because they are either too embarrassed or aren't sure whether what they experience is normal. Please speak out. Help is available.

○ The risk of cancer with heavy periods is tiny. There are many more common causes.

○ Endometriosis is way more than just painful periods. It can cause pain during sex, when going to the toilet and generally throughout the month because you can get scar tissue developing inside your pelvis that can make your organs stick together.

○ PMS and PMDD may be the butt of many jokes in society but they are no laughing matter for many women. It's not in your head, it's real.

○ You can still get pregnant if you have sex during your period. Blood is not a contraceptive, I'm afraid. Unless it makes your man run for the hills, of course.

PART THREE

Sexual Health and Screening

feel this section should be called 'Things that cause the most tears in the gynaecology clinic' – and this is mostly because there isn't enough education about the topics covered here. I don't mind if you cry, as long as you tell me exactly what you're crying about, so that we work it out together. As a doctor, one of the worst feelings is when a patient leaves the room and I don't feel I really got to the bottom of what was bothering them, even if I did address their physical symptoms.

Vaginal discharge gets a bad rap: it's often regarded as a 'symptom' when, in fact, it's the most normal thing and is the reason we all exist, because it helps sperm get to the egg, and produces protective proteins to prevent infection both during and outside of pregnancy. I'm frequently asked about it, and it's important for women to understand what is normal in order to be able to identify when it's not, hence Chapter 6 is devoted to this.

Access to sex education in schools can be patchy, and if you combine the embarrassment of having to listen to your form tutor looking uncomfortable, with everyone giggling and often feeling just as awkward, it's not surprising that people often don't take away much from these sessions. Contraception is not something that is spoken about in many households either, and there is often the fear that talking to teenagers will encourage earlier onset of sexual activity. Therefore, the majority of sex education usually comes from

Chinese whispers, social media and women's magazines, all of which I've found to be hideously inaccurate at times, so Chapter 7 should help to address this.

Then there are sex-related accidents – what if you have one of those? And what happens when you have an abortion? Chapter 8 will give you the answers to the many whispered questions I've been asked, which you definitely don't want to get from Dr Google for fear of being swamped by horror stories and pro-life propaganda.

The final chapter in this section will focus on cervical screening (smear testing), which is something that I researched during my Ph.D. Contrary to popular belief, this is not a 'cervical-cancer test', but the number-one way to prevent a cervical cancer. I see so many women who don't understand what a smear test is for, and also some who come to the colposcopy clinic (where you are investigated if you have an abnormal smear) who are absolutely distraught, convinced that they have cancer because they don't understand their test results. Most of the online information about this is dull and unappealing to the young women who need to come for the test. But by increasing awareness, we can increase the number of women who attend their screening, which will, ultimately, save lives. The HPV vaccine is one of the most exciting developments in this field and also needs to be talked about because it's had some unwarranted bad press, resulting in declining vaccination rates, which means girls are not being protected against a totally preventable cancer.

CHAPTER 6

Vaginal discharge

*'I'm really worried about vaginal discharge . . .
it's happening all the time, but it keeps changing.
Sometimes it's white, sometimes yellow and
sometimes it's really clear and stringy.
And there's SO much of it!'*

Far from worrying, what this patient is describing to me is a completely healthy, or what we call 'physiological' discharge. The word physiological can be defined as 'a characteristic of the normal functioning of a living organism'. And vaginal discharge is so normal a characteristic in humans that it's not only the reason that you exist, but also the reason that you don't have a dusty vagina. Stick with me here . . .

Particular types of vaginal discharge can be a warning sign, but in order to recognise that something is abnormal, you first need to understand what is normal. So now that we've clarified that it is normal to have discharge (actually, about 2–5ml per day), let's talk about how it changes throughout your menstrual cycle, depending on the fluctuations in female hormones, what it does and what can suggest something has gone wrong.

Discharge: the circle of life

As we discussed in Chapter 3 (see page 27), Day 1 of your cycle is the day your period starts, and as the bleeding stops, there may be very little discharge because of low levels of oestrogen and progesterone, often resulting in a dry, irritated feeling. It's probably as close as you'll get to feeling like a post-menopausal woman, so remember what you've got to look forward to. Thankfully, hormone levels start to rise, and discharge becomes thicker and then creamier in consistency and is usually white, but it can have a yellowish or greyish tinge.

As we head on to around two weeks after your period started, it's time for ovulation, which is when the ovaries decide it's time to evict an egg or two in the hope of them meeting the sperm of their dreams. At this time, vaginal discharge becomes very thin and watery, and then stretchy, with an egg-white consistency; there can also be a surprising amount, to the point where you may need to wear a panty liner. This type of discharge seems to cause the greatest level of confusion. The oral contraceptive Pill works by stopping ovulation, so if you're using this form of contraception, you're unlikely to experience this type of discharge. I see hordes of women who have stopped taking the Pill after many years and aren't used to this type of ovulation discharge and are really worried it's something abnormal. But it's not. I always reassure them that it's a real sign their body is working normally. However, it is also a sign that you need to either 1. stock up on condoms or 2. schedule date night, whichever way you are inclined on the pregnancy front. Because this type of discharge, as I boldly stated at the start of this chapter, is the reason we exist. It allows sperm to swim up through the cervix into the uterus (or the womb) and fertilise an egg.

A patient who was trying to get pregnant once asked me to

check whether she was producing ovulation discharge. She thought she was, but her fertility tracking app told her she would be ovulating in five days' time, so she couldn't understand how she was making ovulation discharge and was convinced that she must be wrong and the app right. In fact, it was the other way around: the app was wrong, and she was right. My patient clearly knew herself better than the algorithm did, so getting to know your own body can eventually become more accurate than an app will ever be.

Shortly after ovulation, due to falling oestrogen and rising progesterone levels, the discharge becomes very thick and sticky and even the Mo Farahs of the sperm world aren't going to stand a chance of getting through that stuff. It makes a thick plug in the cervix as a way of protecting the uterine cavity from infections in the hope that an egg was fertilised. And if the sperm–egg dating game didn't go so well, your period starts and the cycle repeats itself.

Why do I have vaginal discharge?

As well as ensuring the continuity of the human race, vaginal discharge has many other important roles. When I perform colposcopy (See Chapter 10), I use a microscope with a camera attached to a screen, so that the patient can see what I'm doing during the examination to look at their cervix and the top of their vagina. I love to entertain and educate my patients during their colposcopy, also as a way of keeping them calm, and this usually starts with 'Dr Mitra's guided vagina tour'. Invariably, the first thing they will notice is the discharge, which can often obscure the view:

'Oh my gosh, what's that white stuff?'

'Oh, that's vaginal discharge,' I explain.

'Urgh, that's disgusting! Why is it there? Do I have an

infection?' is the usual response – at which point I take great pleasure in explaining why this 'disgusting' blob of mucus is a normal, healthy thing.

Firstly, discharge contains antibodies and small proteins called antimicrobial peptides that we sometimes refer to as 'natural antibiotics'. They have been shown to protect against sexually transmitted infections, and other bugs that want to wreak havoc, causing things like thrush and bacterial vaginosis. But we also have good bacteria in the vagina, just as we see in the gut, and the vaginal bacterial community is known as the vaginal microbiome. The word microbiome seems to have become a wellness buzzword. And arguably, the human microbiome (the term used to describe the bacterial population that reside in the body) is one of the most exciting areas of science and medicine to be discovered this century. Loads of new research suggests the vaginal microbiome is also pivotal to immune protection of the vagina and upper genital tract, and probably plays a huge role in female health and disease. *Lactobacillus* are the main healthy bacteria here.

But discharge has two other, unexpected functions. Number one, it prevents chafe, and number two, it stops your vagina from getting dusty. I'm honestly not joking. Discharge acts as a lubricant to stop friction and irritation, and also provides a way of helping the dead cells from the vagina, cervix and uterus to make their way out into the outside world.

Discharge production: it's more than just arousal

The type of discharge that I've been talking about is largely made by the glands of the cervix. But there's also a second kind of discharge: the kind that is made during sexual arousal. An increased blood flow to the vulva and vagina occurs as a normal reaction to arousal, which causes a small amount of fluid called 'transudate' to leak through the vaginal walls. The Skene's and Bartholin's glands that sit near the entrance to the vagina also release fluid and together these make the sticky discharge that ensures lubrication to protect the vulval and vaginal tissues from friction and irritation during penetration. The Skene's glands are the female version of the prostate gland and are thought to be the source of the elusive 'female ejaculation' that some women report, although not as often as the porn industry might lead you to believe.

The amount of discharge that you experience related to arousal is dictated by psychological, as well as hormonal factors, which is why you can suddenly start to feel a wetness within minutes if you are thinking about something that turns you on, or you're engaging in foreplay with your partner. You'll often feel drier just before and just after your period, due to the relatively low levels of oestrogen and progesterone, and this can also lead to a decreased blood supply to the area, and less discharge being produced by the Skene's and Bartholin's glands, even if you're as turned on as you could ever be. It may be frustrating, but it's normal, and there's no shame in using a bit of lubricant to make sex a little more comfortable and enjoyable at those times. If you are going to use lube, I would recommend something plain, and not anything tingly or 'self-heating' because that could cause more irritation, since your vagina and vulva are a bit more sensitive to irritation during their drier spells.

Causes of abnormal discharge

Having said that discharge is normal and healthy, not all discharge is created equal, and it's important to know when something is abnormal.

WHEN YOU SMOKE, YOUR VAGINA SMOKES TOO

Smoking is most often associated with lung-related diseases, but nicotine and its metabolites have been found in the vaginal discharge of smokers, as well as that of women exposed to passive smoking.[1] Smoking is known to have anti-oestrogenic effects, which can cause women to go through an early menopause,[2] have osteoporosis,[3] as well as vaginal dryness and higher rates of bacterial vaginosis.[4]

All these complications, among others, seem like pretty good reasons to stop smoking in my opinion. However, this was not a view shared by the boyfriend of a patient I met in clinic a few months ago. She was referred by her GP with guess what? Vaginal dryness and recurrent bacterial vaginosis. I took a thorough history, which I completed in the way that is taught at medical schools worldwide, including asking whether the patient smokes (although I could smell cigarette smoke on both of them as soon as they walked into the room). Before I could even finish the question, her boyfriend jumped down my throat. He began ranting about how all doctors cared about was lecturing people about smoking. He showed no signs of stopping, and his girlfriend, who was now almost curled into a ball in her chair, crying silently, seemed to be shifting away from him and towards me, as if she wanted to be protected. He finally stopped ranting, having tried to rationalise her smoking as a way of handling her stressful lifestyle, and he then remained quiet for the rest of the consultation, while I explained to the patient that stopping smoking was probably the best thing she could do for her symptoms and her health in general, along with some other lifestyle modifications that would also help. I'm not one to judge a book by its cover, but the boyfriend didn't really seem like 'a keeper'. Still, knowing my professional boundaries, as she stood up to leave I simply reinforced my message: 'The best advice I can give you is to have a look at the things we talked about that could make your lifestyle a bit healthier; mainly smoking and trying to address the stresses in your life.' I smiled, and she walked out of the door. I hope she made the right decision – not just about the smoking.

Thrush

Also known as vulvovaginal candidiasis or a 'yeast infection', thrush is caused by a yeast called *Candida* that commonly lives in the vagina. Usually, it does so without causing any harm, but under certain conditions it can take over and causes a cottage cheese-like, white/pale yellow/green vaginal discharge, accompanied by vulval and vaginal itching, burning and general irritation. In severe cases, you may even notice a pink-reddish coloured inflammation of the surrounding skin.

It's absolutely fine to use over-the-counter medication from the pharmacy without seeing a doctor, but if it doesn't get better you do need to see someone to confirm it is definitely thrush. Most people tend to prefer the tablets, but if you treat yourself with a vaginal cream or tablet, make sure you read the instruction leaflet because some of these will damage condoms.

I'm often asked if yoghurt works for thrush, and the answer is yes, it's actually been suggested to be as effective as clotrimazole cream[5] (although probably messier), but with an overwhelming number of types of natural yoghurt, I would probably reserve it for times when the dreaded itch starts on a rainy Sunday evening and you'd rather lounge on the sofa than try to find a twenty-four-hour pharmacy.

While the yeast can be passed on during sex, there's no need for your partner to be treated unless they have symptoms because it hasn't been shown to reduce recurrence rates.[6]

Thrush is more common in diabetics, oral contraceptive-Pill users and during pregnancy, due to its association with higher levels of both sugar and oestrogen. Recurrent thrush, defined as three bouts or more in a year, is unfortunately quite common; at least 5 per cent of women get this,[7] and it is another indication to visit your GP to check for undiagnosed diabetes, and also to consider whether you need a long-term anti-yeast medication to reduce the number of episodes you're having. If you're taking the combined Pill, you could discuss switching to a different type of non-oestrogen-containing contraception to see if that helps.

I am asked a lot about probiotics for thrush and I'm a massive fan, much to the surprise of many patients. It's been shown that they can increase cure rates when taken alongside a standard thrush medicine, and also decrease the chance of recurrence in the short term.[8] Whether it is effective as a standalone treatment has not yet been proven, but from my Ph.D. research into the vaginal microbiome, I remain hopeful and don't think there is any harm in trying. I recommend that women with recurrent thrush take a daily probiotic for the long term, and have seen a decrease in the number of episodes in those I've advised to do this. You don't have to use a cream for the bacteria to get to the right place – oral probiotics work perfectly; look for a product containing *Lactobacillus rhamnosus* and *Lactobacillus reuteri* because they're the two species with the greatest amount of clinical evidence behind them.

Bacterial vaginosis (BV)

This can be a distressing infection, which, just like thrush, causes a really irritating discharge that can also be recurrent. It's caused by bacteria, as the name would suggest, and is the overgrowth of various types of 'unhealthy' bacteria that take over the vagina and halt the growth of the healthy *Lactobacillus* (see page 77). The discharge can be thin or creamy in consistency, in varying shades of white, grey, green or yellow, and it has a characteristic smell, often described as 'rotten fish'. Contrary to popular belief, it's not caused by poor hygiene. In fact, excessive hygiene can actually cause it by washing away healthy bacteria, and this is something I've seen countless times. Common sense tells us that if something smells, that's because it's dirty and needs washing. This is absolutely not the case for your vagina.

Many women tend to get it just at the end of or after their period because that's the time when oestrogen levels are at their lowest, which means the *Lactobacillus* don't have much support to grow, so the bad bacteria can break free and take over. This is also the reason we see higher levels in women who have gone through the menopause.[9] Smokers are also known to have higher rates of bacterial vaginosis,[4] and there is no known 'safe' level of smoking, so if BV is a problem for you and you do smoke, quitting is the only way to know if it's going to help you.

There's also a common misconception that BV is a sexually transmitted infection, which it isn't. However, semen does make the vagina less acidic and can slow the growth of healthy *Lactobacillus*, which may be why so many women report getting it after having a lot of sex. Treatment is with antibiotics – either oral tablets or vaginal cream – although recurrence rates are high.[10] Using condoms doesn't seem to help many people in my experience, so what's a girl to do? Well, this is where my beloved probiotics come in. The published evidence isn't as strong as it could be,[11] but (in my opinion) that's because the patients in the studies didn't take the probiotics long term, so most studies have shown good cure rates but still high recurrence. For recurrent bacterial vaginosis you need to continue taking the probiotic long term because there's probably a tiny population of the BV-causing bacteria that live dormant in your vagina, taking over whenever the opportunity presents itself and resulting in further episodes. By feeding your vagina with *Lactobacillus* on a daily basis, you have the best chance of stopping this from happening.

There are also a lot of over-the-counter vaginal creams and 'pH-balancing' products. For every person who says they work there seems to be another who says they are a waste of money and just make a mess, but I don't have a problem with them, and if they work for you, that's fine.

Again, treating your male partner doesn't seem to help either,[12] and not because he has a dirty penis, as one of my patients was once told.

In reality, there are probably a multitude of factors that cause BV that we'll never get to the bottom of, but it does seem that some women are just more likely to get it due to their genes, so if that's you, please don't blame yourself and remember it's not a sign that you or your partner are dirty.

Sexually transmitted diseases

This is a surprisingly infrequent cause of abnormal discharge. Chlamydia is the commonest sexually transmitted bacterial infection in the UK, and doesn't cause any symptoms in 70 per cent of cases, and this is particularly true for women. Gonorrhoea is less common, but also tends to be without symptoms in the majority of infected individuals. However, an STI should be considered and tested for in the case of abnormal discharge because they are relatively common and can have serious side effects. STIs and their complications are covered in Chapter 9.

||||||||||||||||||||||||||||||||||||||||||||

THINGS YOU'VE ALWAYS WANTED TO KNOW, BUT WERE TOO AFRAID TO ASK

What are the things to look out for that suggest something isn't quite right?

If you have discharge associated with any of the following, it's time to go and see a doctor:

- Persistent itching that doesn't go after treatment with over-the-counter thrush cream/tablets
- Blood-stained discharge
- Foul smell – I hate the term 'rotten fish' because it reminds me of the disgusting things that teenage boys talk about in the playground, but it's actually fairly accurate because the chemicals that give the discharge its characteristic smell are similar to those produced by rotting fish/meat
- Abdominal pain

- Pain/burning/stinging on passing urine
- Presence of blisters/ulcers/lumps/bumps on your vulva

How should I clean my vagina?

Quite simply, you shouldn't. Your vagina is self-cleaning. Discharge, containing old cells that need to come away, is one of the ways that it does this and gravity helps it along nicely. There are a lot of feminine-hygiene products on the market, including washes and wipes. While they all claim to be 'kind' and pH-friendly, they're not necessary at all. I see a lot of people who use them for irritation, but, in fact, they cause even more irritation because they wash away the healthy Lactobacillus, stopping it from growing, which is often the reason for the irritation in the first place. The good vaginal bacteria make their way there from the anus, so even vigorous washing on the outside could stop this normal bacterial transfer and make irritation and excessive discharge worse.

Should I steam clean my vagina?

Please don't. This has been suggested by certain celebrities, none of whom have any kind of medical or scientific training. Steam clean your carpets to get rid of bacteria, by all means, but not your vagina, as doing so too will kill bacteria in a non-selective manner: the bad bugs will die, but so too will poor little Lactobacillus – cue more irritation and discharge. And the tissue there is so delicate that the risk of labial burns also doesn't sound worth it to me.

I was once at a market in London and stopped at a stall where a woman was selling a vaginal-steaming seat. She started telling me about how it could cure PCOS, endometriosis, fibroids . . . Her non-evidence-based sales pitch was a lot of hot air and I had to walk away.

Is there any evidence for the Candida diet in preventing thrush?

There is minimal evidence to support the use of the Candida diet – a low-sugar diet containing non-starchy vegetables, non-glutinous grains, fermented foods and a moderate amount of lean protein – for either vaginal thrush, or the overgrowth of Candida in the gut for which it is really intended. The thing that irritates me about this diet is that its creators recommend kicking off with a 'cleanse phase' and they do slightly vilify certain food groups, which turns it into more of a fad for me, but I do appreciate the concept, which focuses around eating lots of fresh vegetables, lean protein and good-quality fats. While a lot of us could probably benefit from decreasing the amount of sugar in our diets, it's only diabetics who would expect to see an increase in the risk of thrush with sugar consumption, since the rest of us can rely on our pancreas to produce insulin to keep our blood sugar under control.

And what about coconut oil?

While we're on the topic of fads, I think coconut oil deserves a mention here too because it has been shown to have anti-Candida activity in lab experiments,[13] and I've even seen websites telling women to use coconut-oil-soaked tampons to treat thrush. There are no human studies to back up such a practice, plus coconut oil seems to have quite broad-spectrum antibacterial activity too, which means it may kill off the good Lactobacillus gang as well as the Candida, so it's not something I would recommend.

||||||||||||||||||||||||||||||||||||||||||

THE GYNAE GEEK'S KNOWLEDGE BOMBS

You may have been surprised to find an entire chapter devoted to vaginal discharge, but as it is the reason you exist and it protects you against disease, while also pro-voking massive anxiety, I think it's a good call. So please do remember the following points:

- It's normal to have vaginal discharge that changes throughout your cycle.
- You need to learn what's normal for you, so that you can work out if something is abnormal.
- Thin, watery, egg-white-like discharge in the middle of the cycle is a healthy sign that you are ovulating.
- Smoking increases your risk of thrush, bacterial vaginosis and vaginal dryness.
- STIs are a rare cause of abnormal discharge and they're often asymptomatic, but they still need to be checked for.

CHAPTER 7

Contraception

Me: *Are you sexually active?*

Patient: *Yes.*

Me: *And what kind of contraception do you use?*

Patient: *None . . .*

Me: *Oh, OK. So are you trying to get pregnant at the moment?*

Patient: (often avoiding eye contact at this point)
No.

We all think: it won't happen to me. But it can. It does. And it will. Especially if you haven't had a decent education when it comes to contraception. If 100 couples have sex on a regular basis for one year, 84 will get pregnant,[14] so if you don't want to, you need to use a reliable method of contraception.

I've seen a huge rise in young, often highly educated women using the withdrawal method because they're sick of taking the Pill, often because the latest 'all natural' wellness trend tells them they shouldn't – yet they've never have any trouble with it before. So in this chapter, I intend to set a few things straight to ensure that you're able to protect yourself with a method that is reliable and acceptable to you.

There is also a tendency to focus on contraception solely in terms of preventing pregnancy, but it's important to remember that it is also a way of preventing sexually transmitted infections, and while they're often easily treated, they can have some rather unpleasant side effects such as infertility and chronic pelvic pain, so being blasé with contraception is definitely not without some potentially serious, long-term complications (see Chapter 9).

Contraception is by no means a luxury item, and the World Health Organization must agree with me because they've included the Pill, injection, implant, ring, Mirena and copper coils, diaphragm and condoms in their 'List of Essential Medicines' – the safest and most effective therapies to meet the essential needs of a healthcare system.[15] With an abundance of options available, there is something for everyone. So without further ado, let's look at a rundown of these, with a summary in the table below.

Hormonal contraception

When the term 'hormonal contraception' is mentioned, we tend to think first of the Pill. While this is indeed the most commonly used type, there are several other forms. So let me take you through them.

The Combined Oral Contraceptive Pill (COCP)

This is the most commonly used contraception in the UK.[16] It contains two active ingredients – a synthetic oestrogen and progesterone – and its main mode of action is to prevent ovulation. So no egg = no fertilisation = no baby.

The Pill is frequently criticised by the media, and unfairly in my opinion. While there are undoubtedly side effects, if you want a really effective contraception, with the added advantage of potentially lighter, less painful periods, improved acne and less PMS, the Pill is for you. For some

THE WITHDRAWAL METHOD: RUSSIAN ROULETTE OR CONTRACEPTION?

The withdrawal method, or *Coitus interruptus*, is thought to be used by 8 per cent of couples as their main form of contraception.[17] (If I was asked to put a figure on it, I would have gone much higher, based on the huge number of women who tell me they use withdrawal in place of a reliable method at least occasionally, if not as their sole method for preventing pregnancy.)

In all honesty, the withdrawal method is like playing Russian roulette, but with a penis instead of a gun. The quoted failure rate is up to 24 per cent and one study showed that 37 per cent of pre-ejaculatory fluid contains healthy, motile sperm[18] (i.e. the type that is ready and willing to brave the river rapids of the vagina and cervix to make it to an egg and fertilise it).

Furthermore, it surely takes the pleasure out of sex?

women it can be a game-changer, enabling them to tolerate life on their period.

Many women tell me they are on the Pill with a hint of shame in their voice, or they say they've been taking it for 'too long', diverting their gaze as if I'm about to tell them they're doing something wrong. So it should be noted that there's no limit to the length of time you can safely use the Pill. Furthermore, there has been a decrease in the number of Pill users in the UK over the last few years,[19] yet the potential health benefits are drastically underplayed by the media, and a large study has shown that using the Pill reduces the risk of bowel, endometrial and ovarian cancers,[20] which are responsible for 29 per cent of all female cancer diagnoses and 18 per cent of female cancer deaths annually;[21,22] and, in fact, the overall cancer risk in women who have ever used the pill is 4 per cent less than in those who have not.[20] Yet few people are aware of these statistics. What they hear instead is that it can increase your risk of breast and cervical cancer – although that risk is low, disappears within five years of stopping it and is still smaller than the potential protective benefits from the three aforementioned cancers, which last at least three decades after stopping.[20]

Side effects

Besides the sexual freedom that the Pill has given us, we cannot underestimate the degree to which it has improved the quality of life of millions of women, who were previously unable to go about their daily lives due to terribly painful or heavy periods, and dreadful PMS. Yet I also come across plenty of people who really hate the Pill, saying they cannot tolerate the side effects: headaches, mood swings, sore breasts and bleeding in between periods.

It's worth giving yourself a good three months to see how you get on with a particular Pill, and just because one doesn't suit you, don't rule it out completely. There are many brands with different doses of each active ingredient, and you may well find one that works for you.

A more serious potential side effect, however, is that of blood clots in the legs (deep-vein thrombosis) or lungs (pulmonary embolism), so anyone with a history of clots should avoid the Pill, along with smokers over the age of thirty-five and high-altitude climbers.

A good friend from medical school once called me saying

CONTRACEPTION: FAILURE RATES, PROS AND CONS

	Type	Failure rate
HORMONAL		
COCP	User-dependent	Perfect use: 1% Typical use: 9%
POP	User-dependent	Perfect use: 1% Typical use: 9%
Contraceptive injection	LARC	1%
Contraceptive implant	LARC	1%
Contraceptive ring	User-dependent	Perfect use: 1% Typical use: 9%
Mirena coil/ Intrauterine system (IUS)/'hormonal coil'	LARC	0.5%
NON-HORMONAL		
Male condom	User-dependent	Perfect use: 2% Typical use: 18%
Female condom	User-dependent	Perfect use: 5% Typical use: 21%
Copper coil/ Intrauterine device (IUD)	LARC	0.5%
Fertility awareness methods	User-dependent	Perfect use: 1% Typical use: 24%
Vasectomy/Male sterilisation	Permanent	0.05%
Female sterilisation	Permanent	0.5%

LARC = long-acting reversible contraceptive. This is a non-user-dependent contraceptive which provides long-term contraception for the duration of use, but it is completely reversible upon removal.
Perfect use = used consistently, as instructed under ideal conditions.

Pros	Cons
○ Decreased menstrual blood flow ○ May reduce PMS symptoms ○ Can be used to delay periods, if desired	○ Needs to be taken daily ○ Diarrhoea, vomiting and certain medications can make it less effective
○ Decreased menstrual blood flow ○ Safe for smokers, over-35s, high BMI	○ Needs to be taken daily ○ Diarrhoea, vomiting and certain medications can make it less effective
○ Lasts 8–13 weeks	○ Cannot be removed/reversed if side effects develop
○ Lasts 3 years but can be removed sooner	○ Requires a small injection and cut in the skin to insert and remove
○ Stays inside for 3 weeks at a time	○ You are required to insert it inside your vagina and remove it yourself
○ Lasts 3 or 5 years but can be removed sooner ○ Lighter, shorter, less painful periods	○ May cause irregular spotting/ bleeding for the first 6–12 months
○ Protect against sexually transmit- ted infection ○ No side effects	○ Risk of slippage/splitting
○ Protect against sexually transmit- ted infection ○ No side effects	○ Not widely available ○ Higher risk of slippage/improper fit compared to male condoms
○ Lasts 5 or 10 years but can be removed sooner	○ Periods may be heavier, longer and more painful
○ Increased awareness of menstrual cycle ○ No side effects	○ Need to avoid sex/use a condom during fertile period
○ No side effects	○ Not easily reversed
○ No side effects	○ Not easily reversed

User-dependent = The failure rate is dependent on how you use it, e.g. do you forget to take your Pill every day? Do you put a condom on halfway through intercourse?
Typical use = used as intended, but taking into account human error and non-ideal conditions of average use.

that she'd read in a magazine that women should stop the Pill every few months to give their bodies a break. This is completely non-evidence-based; plus, stopping and starting on a frequent basis is not recommended because the risk of blood clots is greatest in the first six months of use.

Finally, one of the most common concerns about the Pill is that it may cause weight gain, and we all know that friend/ sister/girl at university who ballooned in size when taking it. However, this has not been proven in a large robust study.[23] The oestrogen component of the Pill might make you retain a bit more water, and may also slightly increase your appetite, but it shouldn't account for anything more than a couple of kilos at most. Ultimately, I think different people react differently to different hormone combinations, so as I said earlier, you can always try an alternative Pill if you do find you've put on a lot of weight.

The main reason for the Pill to fail is forgetting to take it, or taking it too late, but there are a few other factors discussed below. One baffled patient who only saw her boyfriend at weekends could not believe she was pregnant because, as she said, 'Doctor, I *always* remember to take it at the weekend; not so much in the week, but I'm not having sex then.' I must stress that you do need to take it properly the entire month if you want it to work, not just on the days you're planning to use it for contraception.

It probably sounds like I'm being paid to promote the Pill. Trust me though, there is absolutely no #ad/#paidpost/#conflictofinterest going on here. But as someone who has encountered countless heartbroken, confused, scared women who found themselves accidentally pregnant, I truly believe that no woman should ever be made to feel ashamed for wanting to use a reliable form of contraception.

The Progesterone-Only Pill (POP)

This Pill works primarily by thickening the mucus produced by the cervix, so that sperm cannot 'pass GO and collect £200'. It is a popular choice after having a baby because it's suitable for use while breastfeeding, whereas the COCP can interfere with milk production. It's also suitable if you can't take the COCP for other reasons including migraine, high blood pressure, diabetes or smoking. Most notably, it doesn't increase the risk of blood clots,[24] so can be used if you have a higher risk of blood clots or if you happen to be a high-altitude climber. I do hear more women reporting weight gain on the POP, however there is little evidence to suggest a direct link between the two.[25]

After one year, half of users will either have no periods or very infrequent ones as a result,[26] which is a bonus for many.

In my opinion, the main downside of the POP is that it's a little less forgiving compared to the COCP in that it needs to be taken within a three- or twelve-hour window (depending on the type) compared to a twenty-four-hour window for the COCP. It also has a slight tendency to worsen acne.[27]

Contraceptive ring

This is a thin ring that sits at the top of your vagina and slowly releases synthetic oestrogen and progesterone. You can't be shy about inserting your fingers into your vagina for this one because that is how you get it in and out every twenty-one days, after which you leave it out for seven days when you'll have a withdrawal bleed. It works in the same way as the COCP, although it contains lower levels of hormone, which could be appealing to many.

You'll know if it's in the right place because you shouldn't really feel it; if you can, the ring is probably too low down and therefore at risk of falling out. Don't worry – it can't get lost in your vagina, as there's nowhere for it to go. I once spent about fifteen minutes in A&E fishing around for someone's 'lost' contraceptive ring. After a protracted exchange of 'I really can't find it – are you sure you didn't remove it?' and 'It must be there; I definitely didn't take it out', the patient finally recalled having removed it three days earlier.

Side effects are similar to those of the COCP (see page 93). A lot of women love the contraceptive ring because it's a great middle ground between the Pill and something longer-lasting, like the coil, because you only need to think about it twice a month.

The implant

This is a 4cm-long, thin tube that is inserted under the skin of the upper arm, where it will not be seen or felt (unless you start poking around – although playing with it under your skin does not cause extra hormone release and won't make it expire any quicker).

Insertion of the implant involves a small injection of local anaesthetic into the skin, following which a tiny cut is made so that the implant can be inserted using a device that looks like a big needle. The skin will then be closed with Steri-Strips, which can be removed after a few days and you can skip off happily, knowing that the implant will give you 99 per cent protection from pregnancy for three years.

The implant provides contraception by releasing a synthetic progesterone which stops ovulation, keeping the cervical mucus thick and impassable to sperm and the endometrial lining thin to prevent implantation. The latter mechanism is the reason why many users stop having periods.

Removal is similar to insertion: a small nick in the skin (possibly with local anaesthetic) so it can be pulled out and then some Steri-Strips. Side effects are comparable to those with the POP (see page 93).

Depo-Medrone injection

This is most popular among under-eighteens, due to ease of use, because it only needs to be given every twelve weeks.

Compared to other forms of hormonal contraception, there is the most evidence that the injection is linked to weight gain – up to 2kg over a year, and most likely in younger users and those who already have a higher BMI.[25] But it's incredibly effective, so that's the pay-off. It tends to stop periods in about half of users, and the chances of this happening increases with duration of use. However, it's not recommended for use for more than two years because it can cause bone thinning (osteopenia), which can progress to osteoporosis, increasing the risk of fractures (a risk which decreases again after stopping the injection).[28]

Mirena coil

The coil is extremely convenient for people with busy lives. Also known as the 'hormone coil', it releases a synthetic progesterone called levonorgestrel, which thickens cervical mucus, making it very difficult for sperm to reach the uterine cavity to fertilise an egg. It also keeps the uterine lining very thin so in the event of a particularly resilient sperm managing to invade, a subsequently fertilised egg would not be able to implant in the womb to grow into a pregnancy. This ability to keep the lining thin means periods are much lighter, with 20 per cent of women having no periods at all by twelve months, rising to 50 per cent at two years.[29] And this, I must stress, is not an unhealthy side effect; if there's no lining to shed, it's not dangerous that you're not getting a period. This is great news for women with troublesome periods, and I see plenty who are really happy with the results – one of which is that far fewer need hysterectomies these days.[30] It's difficult to predict who will stop having periods, but generally

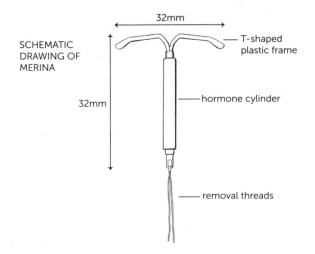

32mm

SCHEMATIC
DRAWING OF
MERINA

32mm

T-shaped
plastic frame

hormone cylinder

removal threads

speaking, the lighter and shorter your periods normally are, the more likely it is that they'll stop completely within a few months of use.[31]

One of the slightly annoying, although temporary side effects of the Mirena coil is that it can cause some irregular bleeding and spotting for the first few months.

We've all heard coil-insertion horror stories, and this is often the reason why some women won't even entertain the suggestion of one. However, I don't know many people who have been unable to have a coil inserted. The whole process only lasts about three minutes. Sometimes local-anaesthetic injections are used, but some women say that's more painful than the coil itself, which is inserted using a thin plastic insertion device (like a very thin drinking straw). I must confess, I have known a few women to faint afterwards, but this was because stimulation of the cervix can cause a drop in blood pressure in a small number of women. You will get a bit of cramping period-like pain afterwards, but it will be gone the following day. And then you can smile in the knowledge that you won't need to think about contraception for the next five years.

A newer hormone coil called Jaydess is now available in the UK. It works on the same principles, although it is marginally smaller at 4mm in height and width, with a central tube that is 1mm smaller in diameter, making insertion slightly easier and less uncomfortable, although it does need to be changed more frequently (every three years) and may be less likely to reduce menstrual flow.[32]

Non-hormonal contraception

Lots of women don't want to use hormonal contraception or have medical reasons for why they shouldn't. For these women, there are several types of non-hormonal contraception options out there.

Condoms

Aside from moving to a convent, condoms are the most effective way of preventing sexually transmitted infections. When it comes to pregnancy prevention, however, they're pretty mediocre. Male condoms are 82 per cent effective with typical use, and this rises to 98 per cent with perfect use (compared, for example, with the Pill, which with typical use is 91 per cent effective and over 99 per cent with perfect use).

So it's all about how you use them. The commonest condom-related errors are putting the condom on upside down and then flipping it over, and putting it on too late in the game.[33] These increase the risk of pregnancy because pre-ejaculatory fluid from the penis, which you might not even notice, can actually contain semen. This is also the reason that you need to be a bit careful about playing around down there if it's starting to get a bit 'juicy', shall we say?

I once had a referral from a GP for a girl who had some pain, a late period and positive pregnancy test. The catch: she'd never had sex before. Oh, OK, I've heard that one before, I thought to myself. But when I went to examine her I realised she was telling the truth. It turned out she'd had a lot of what I might tactfully call 'juicy naked fumbles'. And sure enough, when I scanned her there was a little seven-week-sized pregnancy with a heartbeat. It's not common, but it can happen – so be aware!

Female condoms are much harder to find and much less frequently used as a result. They are also slightly more likely to fail, probably due to the fact that they don't have such a tight fit, and so there's a risk of the penis slipping down the side between the condom and vaginal wall, rather than into the condom itself.

Copper coil

The copper coil has been around for absolutely yonks (since the 1970s, if you're wondering), and there's recently been a renewed interest in it, due to increasing demand for effective, non-hormonal contraception. They are similar in shape and size to the Mirena and can stay in place for five to ten years. The copper on the stem has a toxic effect on the sperm and the egg, although not on the cells of the female reproductive tract.

The main unwanted effect of the copper coil is that your period will usually be heavier[34] and more painful in the first few months, and this is the most common cause for early removal.[35] This is not always properly explained, and it can come as a shock to a lot of women, particularly if they're changing from the Pill, which has probably made their periods lighter. Therefore, I wouldn't recommend it to you if you already find your periods heavy or painful.

Removal, should you want it, is pretty simple, and not anywhere near as involved as insertion. You can't do it yourself though. You need a speculum examination and we use a small pair of graspers to hold the strings and pull it down. The copper coil can also be used as emergency contraception up to five days after unprotected sex has taken place (see Chapter 8).

Fertility-awareness methods

This is also known as the rhythm method or periodic abstinence. The aim is to identify the fertile period during your cycle (see pages 101–2 and 161–2) and abstain from intercourse during that time (which is when you're programmed to have the highest sex drive since the workings of your menstrual cycle are all about trying to get pregnant). If you're using this method, you either need to be really strict about not having sex on your fertile days or use condoms at that time. Also, bear in mind that you may inaccurately predict your day of ovulation due to matters beyond your control, such as stress, illness, altered sleeping patterns; this is why the failure rate is around 24 per cent (so if you and three friends all use this method for a year, one will get pregnant).

This method may be suitable for you if you're someone who has a very regular menstrual cycle and you become aware of the fertile cues such as a change in vaginal discharge and cervical positioning (the position and texture of the cervix change through the month; with careful teaching it is possible to learn how to detect these changes). But I cannot overemphasise the fact that it requires a great deal of patience and isn't really something you can learn from a quick read of a web page.

Contraceptive apps

We use our mobile phones for almost everything: ordering takeaways, checking the weather, sending emails. But can we also use them as contraception? Some people think so, although the apps in question are not currently recommended by the NHS because the preliminary data suggests most are not effective enough.[36] Nevertheless, I am frequently bombarded with questions about them, especially given the abundance of social-media influencers being paid to advertise them.

The app aims to learn your menstrual cycle and you help it to determine your fertile period by strictly logging daily body temperature, enabling it to detect the 0.3°C temperature increase that occurs at ovulation. Using this information, the app works out whether you are fertile or not and therefore tells you if it's safe to have sex or not. Studies suggest a 7.5 per cent failure rate using these apps.[37] So why would the app get it wrong? Well, there are many reasons, including not taking your temperature at the same time every day, having a fever due to illness, being in a different time zone that affects your circadian rhythm or you just happen to ovulate on a day the app didn't predict (the latter can be surprisingly common). Or maybe you just have an irregular cycle, making it really tricky for the app to learn.

This method is particularly unsuitable for people with PCOS, as they may have very long cycles (e.g. one period every two to three months) with lots of LH surges (this is what causes that temperature spike the app is looking for to help it predict your fertile time). Lots of LH surges = unpredictable temperature rises = lots of red days = you not being very happy with the app.

The bottom line is that if you ovulate earlier than expected and you've had unprotected sex within five days, you are at risk of pregnancy because the rise in temperature only happens on the actual day of ovulation and sperm can live in the body for five days. Therefore, the app will be late in realising it's your fertile window and you may already have had unprotected sex. You'll still need to use condoms during the fertile window or avoid having sex altogether, which doesn't appeal to a lot of the people I've spoken to.

My view here is that it's OK if you wouldn't be devastated if you got pregnant. Conversely, you can use it to help you plan for a pregnancy (see Chapter 11).

Sterilisation

The number of men and women undergoing sterilisation has steadily fallen over the last decade, which is probably due to the increasing use of other long-term contraceptives like the coil.[19] Male sterilisation is the most effective, and can be done under local anaesthetic, so although you can't quite regard 'the Snip' as a lunchtime procedure, there is minimal risk or downtime. It's theoretically reversible, although reversal isn't available on the NHS and isn't always successful.[38]

Female sterilisation is a bit more of an undertaking and was referred to as 'HMS point-of-no-return' by a Fijian obstetrician I worked with on my medical-school elective. It requires laparoscopic (keyhole) surgery under general anaesthetic to cut the tubes or apply clips to block them. It is also something that we occasionally do at the time of a planned Caesarean section, although it is good practice for you to have discussed it with your obstetrician during the pregnancy; because of its permanent nature, it must not be an impulse decision. It's our duty to give you plenty of time to consider if it really is the right option for you, rather than making an off-the-cuff decision on the day of the delivery when you have a million other things going through your

CONTRACEPTION AND TRAVEL

- **COCP** If changing time zones you'll need to try and adjust the time you take it to be similar to when you are at home – so, for example, 7 a.m. in London would be 2 a.m. in Miami. It's better to take it earlier rather than later, so 10 p.m. in Miami instead. Remember to keep mobile, wear compression stockings and stay well hydrated on the flight to reduce the risk of blood clots. It's not recommended at altitudes greater than 4,500 metres (this includes Mount Kilimanjaro so it's not just extreme explorers that need to consider this). Consider switching to another method before your trip.
- **POP** Be mindful of the three- or twelve-hour time window for taking it. That can get tricky with jet lag. Don't forget about the chance of getting a tummy bug if you're going somewhere exotic, so if you're going somewhere remote, or don't want a 'Bridget Jones in the pharmacy'-type scene, you may want to think about taking some emergency contraception in the form of the morning-after Pill (see page 111).
- **Fertility awareness methods/apps** Timing of ovulation may be incredibly difficult to predict when you're working with jet lag, or even just a change of schedule, so it may be worthwhile considering a different type of contraception while you're travelling and for some time after you get back until you think your cycle is back into the swing of things.
- **Contraceptive injection, implant, both types of coil, condoms and sterilisation** These are not affected by travel in any way.

mind and are probably so fed up of being pregnant at that precise point in time that the idea of another child is not something you can begin to consider. You'll notice I referred to 'its permanent nature'; it is sometimes possible to have a reversal done in a private hospital, although again it isn't always successful, and comes with a much higher risk of ectopic pregnancy.

|||||||||||||||||||||||||||||||||||||||||

THINGS YOU'VE ALWAYS WANTED TO KNOW, BUT WERE TOO AFRAID TO ASK

Will hormonal contraception decrease my chance of getting pregnant in the future?

Hormonal contraception is completely reversible and does not have a long-term impact on fertility after you stop using it. Pill users do not take any longer to get pregnant after stopping, compared to condom users.[39] The same is true for the contraceptive ring, implant,[40] Mirena and copper coils.[41]

The contraceptive injection is the one to avoid if you're planning on getting pregnant straight after using it. Fertility can take some time to return with this because the drug will take a while to dissolve away completely after the initial three months for which it is guaranteed as a contraceptive. Fertility should usually return by about ten months, but can take up to almost two years.[42] There is no risk to fertility in the long term, so using it as a teenager won't stop you getting pregnant in your mid-twenties, for example.

Some hormonal contraception will stop periods in some users and not others, but there's no evidence to suggest that those who don't have periods on the contraception will take longer to get pregnant than those who did.

Does the Pill cause depression?

No one is entirely sure at the moment. We all know someone who has said the Pill caused them to feel 'moody and irrational' or like 'a total monster', but a real minority become clinically depressed or anxious.

A study of over a million Danish women caused quite a stir when it was published in 2016, due to its conclusion that users of the COCP, POP, contraceptive patch, ring and hormonal coil were more likely to be diagnosed with depression. But on closer inspection, the statistics showed that only about 1 in 200 women who used hormonal contraception developed depression, who might not have developed it otherwise.[43] A further study of almost a million Swedish women found only the POP, and not the COCP to be associated with depression.[44] And numerous other studies have failed to find any link at all.[45, 46] However, the most consistent finding is the suggestion that women with a history of depression and mental-health problems are most likely to experience a negative effect from the Pill.

There aren't any good studies examining whether stopping hormonal contraception can improve mood. And remember that not everyone is using it to prevent pregnancy, and it has been shown that women using it for non-contraceptive purposes were more likely to report depressive symptoms,[47] which may be due to the higher risk of depression associated with their underlying disease (such as endometriosis or PCOS).

In my opinion, the most important thing that we can take away from these studies is that there is certainly an interplay between female hormones and mental health, but we can't be sure who it affects and to what extent. Ultimately, it may be difficult to ever truly determine whether hormonal contraception causes mental-health problems, because of the fact there are so many confounding factors and it's unlikely to be the same mechanism for everyone.

This confirms that choosing contraception requires a tailored approach, one-to-one with a healthcare professional, to decide the best type for you, and that you shouldn't feel afraid to mention mood symptoms as well as physical ones at your follow-up appointments. Anyone who is worried that there may be a connection between their mental health and their contraception should discuss this with their GP or contraception provider, switching either to another type of Pill (different active ingredients may have different effects) or another reliable method. The psychological impact that unintended pregnancy can also bring should not be underestimated.[48,49]

Is there anything that can stop the Pill from working?

Anything that stops the COCP/POP from being absorbed or speeds up its metabolism will decrease drug levels within the blood, which will increase the likelihood of unplanned pregnancy. These include:

- diarrhoea and vomiting (check the packet instructions for accurate advice)
- detox teas – this is almost like giving yourself diarrhoea; everything goes quicker through your bowel, so there's less time for absorption
- charcoal – it non-selectively binds drugs, chemicals, toxins . . . and your Pill; there are no clear health benefits from drinking charcoal lattes/smoothies, etc., so if you don't want a surprise in nine months, I suggest finding another Instagrammable drink
- herbal and prescribed medication (including specific epilepsy medication, antiviral, antibiotics and St John's

wort); don't forget to tell anyone who is prescribing/
recommending medication or supplements that you're
taking the Pill, and check with your doctor/pharmacist
if you're not sure.

||||||||||||||||||||||||||||||||||||||

THE GYNAE GEEK'S KNOWLEDGE BOMBS

There is no better way to choose contraception than face-to-face with a healthcare professional. We are so lucky to have so many options, with something for everyone, but remember that they all have their side effects and downsides – no one method is perfect.

These are my key takeaway points from this chapter:

- The withdrawal method is not a reliable form of contraception.
- The Pill has health benefits that aren't sexy enough for the tabloids to talk about.
- Hormonal contraceptives do not harm fertility in the long term and you don't need to take a break from the Pill 'to give your body a rest'.
- The copper coil is in vogue right now, and highly effective, but remember it can make your periods heavier and more painful, especially at the start.
- Many contraceptives work by decreasing or stopping your periods, which in this case is not unhealthy.

CHAPTER 8

Emergency contraception and termination of pregnancy

'I had unprotected sex last night, but I've taken the emergency contraceptive pill, so I'm scared to take it again because I've heard it makes you infertile.'

Just over half of pregnancies in the UK are planned, with 17 per cent being totally unplanned and the remainder being what I would call 'happy accidents'.[50] Emergency contraception (EC) or post-coital contraception is a method used to prevent pregnancy after unprotected intercourse. It does not protect in any way against STIs. It's estimated that 20 per cent of pregnancies end in abortion in the UK, and almost 1 in 10 of women aged 16–49 years uses emergency contraception annually,[51] most commonly in the under-twenties age group.[19]

From my discussions with patients, I think that emergency contraception is underutilised due to a lack of awareness as to exactly what it is, how it works and when it should be taken, as well as the taboo surrounding its use.[51] You may not want or plan to take it, but it's really important to know it is an option.

There is one case that sticks in my head from when I was working in an Urgent Care Centre in a central London A&E

department. A seventeen-year-old girl came in to see me late one Sunday night, requesting emergency contraception. She told me she'd had unprotected sex on the Friday night, and when I asked her why she had waited so long to come in she said she hadn't realised there was such thing as emergency contraception until she was chatting to her friend that evening. Recognising that this girl clearly had very little access to decent sex education, I asked if she had any other more general questions. She looked up at me and asked, 'What do I do if he won't wear a condom?' My heart sank. Not only because a seventeen-year-old, living in central London of all places, was unaware of emergency contraception, but because I could spend all night educating her, but it wouldn't do a damned thing to educate the boys she was sleeping with about the importance of contraception. I did my best to try and empower her to have the courage to demand future condom use, and prescribed the morning-after Pill, along with an anti-sickness tablet (because it is known to cause nausea).

Understanding emergency contraception

An ancient Greek gynaecologist Soranos of Ephesus first described an emergency contraceptive technique which involved the female holding her breath and pulling away from her partner at the time of ejaculation, followed by trying to provoke a sneezing fit, swabbing out her vagina and drinking a glass of cold water. While I have not found any studies reporting the success rates of this technique, there are several more scientifically based methods available today, which are detailed below – two types of hormonal pill and the copper coil.

More than just the 'morning-after Pill'

'Morning-after Pill' (MAP) is a bit of a misnomer because it can actually be used up to three or five days 'after', depending on which type you use. However, the longer you leave it, the less effective it is. Levonelle (Levonogestrel) is the 'old-fashioned' version which can be used up to three days after unprotected sex, while the newest Pill, ellaOne (Ullipristal acetate), may be slightly more effective and can be taken up to five days after. It's estimated that there is an 8 per cent pregnancy risk following a single episode of unprotected sex. After taking Levonelle this may go down to 2.2 per cent, and after ellaOne it's as low as 1.4 per cent.[52] The tablets work by preventing ovulation. If you've ovulated within 24 hours of having sex, and are thus within your fertile window, it can still be taken, but it's unclear whether it does work then and, if it does, what the mechanism actually is. Your next period after taking either MAP may be early or late and is usually heavier than normal. If there is bleeding, but it is incredibly light, I would suggest taking a pregnancy test to check it really is a period and not an implantation bleed, which is spotting or light bleeding that can occur as the pregnancy implants into the womb lining.

In the UK, the MAP can be bought over the counter by anyone over the age of sixteen without a prescription or dispensed by a pharmacist with special prescribing rights to females of any age. This was a controversial move made in 2001 to increase access to emergency contraception and it has not subsequently been shown to increase usage or rates of unprotected sex as was feared.[53]

Note: a word of warning – if you use ellaOne and you're on the Pill, you'll need to use condoms for the next two weeks because it makes the Pill less effective.

Copper coil

While it is only used in about 7 per cent of women requiring emergency contraception, the remainder using the hormonal pill,[19] the copper coil is actually the best form of emergency contraception, being shown in a large study to be 99.91 per cent effective.[54] Not only is it toxic to sperm, thus killing it before it can fertilise an egg, it also prevents implantation. The main advantage is that after being fitted as an emergency, the coil can be left in place as regular contraception for the next five to ten years, depending on the brand, although it can also be removed after your next period if you don't want ongoing contraception. You've also got a longer window for use – up to five days after unprotected sex, or five days after the earliest possible day you could have ovulated, so you'd need to know when your last period was if you use the latter rule. You may be given antibiotics at the time of insertion if there's a risk you may have an STI as well, which could be pushed further up by putting in the coil. **Note**: the hormone coil cannot be used for emergency contraception.

Termination of pregnancy

Termination of pregnancy, also called induced abortion, is a very sensitive topic that is frequently the subject of various moral, religious, political and social opinions. In this section I want to give you the unbiased medical facts, to which you can then apply your own beliefs to decide what you might do if ever faced with such a difficult decision. (**Note**: The term 'abortion' can be confusing. In some countries 'spontaneous abortion' can be used to refer to miscarriage; the spontaneous loss of pregnancy before 24 weeks gestation. In the UK and throughout this book the term 'abortion' is used to refer

UK LAW

The 1967 Abortion Act allows abortion to be carried out in England, Scotland and Wales before twenty-four weeks of pregnancy if there is a risk to the woman's life, the physical or mental health of her or her existing children or if the baby has severe abnormalities. So it's not just unwanted pregnancies that end in abortion. About 2 per cent of terminations per year in the UK are due to abnormalities of the baby,[55] and watching a couple go through this is probably one of the most heartbreaking parts of my job.

It is also legal to perform a termination after twenty-four weeks in a number of rare circumstances, again relating to danger to the mother or her unborn child. None of these circumstances applies in Northern Ireland, where any kind of abortion at any gestation is still illegal, and consequently several thousand women per year come to England, Wales and Scotland to have an abortion.

In addition, the partner of the woman is neither able to give consent to or refuse/prevent a termination.

to the medical process to actively end a pregnancy before normal childbirth.)

About 20 per cent of pregnancies in England and Wales end in abortion, and while many people assume that these are just teenagers, there has actually been a decline in the number of abortions in women under thirty and a rise in women over that age in England over the last decade.[55]

How do I arrange a termination?

You need to go and see your GP, who will discuss with you your reasoning for wanting a termination. They're not being nosy – it's because they want to ensure you've considered all the options and have come to the appropriate decision for you, and also because they have to sign a legal document to confirm you meet one of the legal criteria above (see page 113). This document will then be given to you to take to the hospital or clinic where you will have the abortion. There, you will have a consultation with another doctor, who will add their own signature to say they agree to the abortion. The aim is for women to be offered this second consultation within five days of being referred by the GP and for the abortion to be completed within three weeks of this.

Being referred to an abortion provider does not automatically mean you have to go through with the procedure and you can change your mind at any time up until you receive the medication or have an operation. So even if you're not sure, it's best not to delay going to speak to your GP. Although you shouldn't rush to make the decision, generally speaking the earlier in the pregnancy that you have a termination the safer it is.

The following are also required:

- **Written consent** You will need to sign a consent form confirming that you agree to the procedure and that you have been told about the risks; you should be given a copy of this to take home.
- **Screening for sexually transmitted infections** About 10 per cent of women having a termination are known to have chlamydia infection, and this can result in infections after the termination.
- **A blood test** This is needed to check your haemoglobin,

to ensure you're not anaemic because you will lose some blood, regardless of which type of termination you have. It also checks your blood type, because if you are Rhesus negative (a type of blood antigen), you will need an injection of anti-D to prevent you making antibodies which could attack a future pregnancy.

o **An ultrasound scan** This is to check how far along you are because this may dictate the type of abortion you are offered, and also to confirm the pregnancy is actually in the uterus. You won't be made to look at the screen or to hear a heartbeat. Anyone who tells you they can do a termination but doesn't plan to do a scan beforehand should prompt you to run for the hills. I can't stress enough the importance of going through the proper channels to a properly regulated clinic. You might find other clinics advertised on the internet, and it is possible to have an abortion through a private provider, but they should still follow these mandatory regulations.

Every few months I will admit someone to hospital with acute pain following a termination in an unlicensed clinic when the woman is subsequently found to have an ectopic pregnancy (where the pregnancy implants outside of the womb, usually in the fallopian tube). The last time this happened, the patient, who was writhing around in pain and clammy from the internal bleeding she was experiencing, said to me, 'But it looked clean and they asked me to sign a form, so I thought it would be OK.' We rushed her straight from A&E to theatre and removed her fallopian tube, as well as the litre and a half of blood that had been slowly trickling into her abdomen after the tube burst. The illegal abortion had almost cost her her life. You may be shocked that such a thing could happen in a country where we have relatively good access to termination services, but it will continue to do so unless we become more aware of the potential risks of going to someone who is not regulated.

Medical abortion

Just over half of all terminations in the UK are carried out using medication.[55] A tablet called mifepristone is initially taken, which blocks progesterone with an aim to signal to the body that the pregnancy is ending. In some people, this results in a little bit of bleeding. Between twenty-four and forty-eight hours later, another tablet called misoprostol is given. This is either swallowed, left to dissolve under the lip or put inside the vagina. This will cause the uterus to start to contract and the cervix to open up. It may feel like very strong period pains. Ibuprofen has been found to be the most effective painkiller while undergoing a medical abortion.[56] Misoprostol can also cause vomiting, so anti-sickness tablets may be given at the same time. Bleeding will usually start within the hour and the pregnancy should be passed about six hours later. It will be heavy with some clots about the size of fifty-pence piece and can continue like that for two to three days.

I'm often asked, 'What will I see coming out?' I've even been called down to A&E at 4 a.m. to examine the contents of a small Tupperware container because a frantic patient who had undergone a medical termination had no idea that there would be anything more than just blood coming out. At five to six weeks pregnant, it will mainly be blood with some small whiteish/grey fleshy pieces. Later on, the pregnancy will often fall out in a white- or grey-coloured sac, the size of which depends on how far along you are. You may see a tiny embryo, but even at nine weeks, the commonest time to have a medical abortion, it's only about 2.5cm long, so you often don't see it due to the heavy bleeding.

In the case of medical abortion after twenty-one weeks, medication must be injected into the foetus. This is to stop the heartbeat prior to you being given the medication, so that it is not born alive. The injection must be administered through your tummy, while the doctor scans to ensure it goes into the correct place. Before twenty-one weeks the baby would not be expected to be born alive.

The advantage of a medical abortion is that you can do it at home and no sedation or general anaesthetic are needed. If you are over twelve to thirteen weeks pregnant, you are usually kept in hospital because you are likely to bleed more and the sac or the placenta may become stuck, requiring urgent medical attention, but we always aim to give women their own room and bathroom where possible.

Note: you may come across websites selling 'home-abortion kits', including both mifepristone and misoprostol. No matter how genuine and 'above board' these websites look, *please don't ever* be tempted to buy from them. They are illegal and for good reason; you don't know whether the tablets you are getting are genuine and you need to be assessed by a doctor before you can safely have these medications prescribed.

Surgical abortion

This can be carried out under general anaesthetic (being put to sleep), under sedation (using intravenous medication to relax you, but you're still awake and may not remember the procedure) or while you are completely awake with a local anaesthetic to numb your cervix. The procedure will be performed on a surgical bed with your legs placed up in stirrups. Prior to the operation you may be given a misoprostol tablet, which is either taken orally or put into the vagina, to soften the cervix to make it easier to insert the suction tube that is used to remove the pregnancy tissue. The procedure itself takes about ten to fifteen minutes, but you will spend at least four to five hours at the hospital or clinic because of the time needed to prepare, including transporting you to theatre, inserting a needle to give you medication and to put you to sleep if you're having a general anaesthetic, and also the time needed for observation afterwards. At after fourteen to fifteen weeks of pregnancy, a surgical termination becomes a little trickier, requiring the cervix to be opened up a lot wider and a pair of forceps used to remove it, along with the placenta. It needs to be done under general anaesthetic and takes longer, with a slightly higher risk of bleeding.

The main advantage of a surgical abortion is that it is completed with fewer visits to the hospital and you will see less blood, but you will still bleed like a heavy period afterwards.

Aftercare

You should be given information about where you can go to seek 24/7 help if you feel unwell after an abortion, as well as a report to show to another healthcare provider, so that they can understand what kind of treatment you have had, although not necessarily why, in order for them to offer you safe ongoing care. The risk of infection is about 10 per cent and you may be given antibiotics at the time of the procedure or to take home with you. A fever, foul-smelling discharge and heavy bleeding are all signs of an infection, and I see these regularly in A&E. You will bleed afterwards because the thickened lining of the womb needs to fall away, which it will do for up to two weeks as the pregnancy hormone levels are dropping. The bleeding will be like a period, but may be heavier than you are used to, and sometimes with small blood clots. This is normal, but you should go to A&E if you are changing pads more frequently than every thirty minutes for two to three hours, or if it's making you feel unwell. Pads are preferable to tampons because they allow the blood and any remaining tissue to escape more freely.

You can expect to have a period within six weeks of a termination. If you don't, you must take a pregnancy test. The rate of ongoing pregnancy is less than 1 per cent, but it does happen. I once treated a patient who'd had a surgical termination at nine weeks and then went to her GP over two months later, reporting feeling bloated. She was found to have an ongoing, healthy pregnancy of about twenty weeks. She actually decided to continue with it in the end. The medication used for termination is not known to cause any long-term risk to babies exposed to it. However, if you find the pregnancy test is positive, you will need to undergo further treatment if you still don't want to be pregnant.

It's normal to feel upset, ashamed, anxious that you've made the wrong decision and even grief, but abortion is not shown to increase the risk of serious future mental-health problems. Please do go and seek help though, if you are struggling.

||||||||||||||||||||||||||||||||||||||||||||

THINGS YOU'VE ALWAYS WANTED TO KNOW, BUT WERE TOO AFRAID TO ASK

Is there a limit to how many times I can take the morning-after Pill?

No, but if you're taking it often, you are clearly in need of a reliable regular contraception, so you should read Chapter 7, and then pay a visit to your GP or a sexual-health clinic.

Levonelle can be taken more than once in a menstrual cycle, but ellaOne cannot. It's not dangerous to take the morning-after Pill several times in a lifetime, but it could result in some frustrating disruption to your menstrual cycle because it works by preventing ovulation.[57] One girl once told me she used the morning-after Pill most months because she didn't want to take the Pill due to the hormones involved. This is not medically advised, and it's a false economy because the morning-after Pill contains a large dose of hormones. And, as you will know from Chapter 7, there are several non-hormonal contraceptives available.

Does emergency contraception cause abortion?

It is a commonly held belief that emergency contraception causes abortions, but it's not correct.[51] Fertilisation can take up to twenty-four hours and implantation begins about five days later, being completed between eight and eighteen days following fertilisation. In 2002, a judicial review concluded that life begins at implantation, therefore anything that either prevents ovulation, fertilisation or implantation is not regarded as an abortion by UK law.

Do bear in mind also that at least 50 per cent of naturally fertilised eggs do not implant in any case.[58] However, if you feel strongly that life does, in fact, begin at fertilisation and you do not want to get pregnant, then you do need to make sure you're using a reliable form of contraception to avoid getting into such a conundrum.

Do abortions affect future fertility?

The short answer is no. Neither medical nor surgical abortion is shown to decrease your chances of getting pregnant in the future.[59] This is also evidenced by the fact that every year, over one third of women having an abortion have had at least one previously.[55]

In the past, surgical termination was performed using a sharp scraper called a 'curette', and this was known to be associated with the formation of adhesions which cause the walls of the uterus to stick together. This is called Asherman's syndrome and is very rare these days because the plastic suction tube that is used today is much more gentle and less traumatic for the walls of the uterus.

Women requesting a termination are more likely to have a sexually transmitted infection, such as chlamydia, and this can affect fertility by causing internal scarring. However, this is not directly related to the termination itself, but to the act of unprotected sex that exposes you to both the risk of pregnancy and an STI.

What are the risks of an abortion?

An abortion does carry certain risks, including:

- incomplete abortion, where small pieces of tissue may be left inside and can cause bleeding and infection
- ongoing pregnancy
- infection
- need for blood transfusion
- uterine perforation (where a hole is made in the wall of the uterus) – this can only happen with a surgical abortion, not with medication.

||||||||||||||||||||||||||||||||||||||||||||||

THE GYNAE GEEK'S KNOWLEDGE BOMBS

Emergency contraception and abortion are both quite taboo subjects, and I find the information online can be misleading or prejudiced. I think it's extremely important for women to be aware of the options and, as I said at the start of this chapter, it is based solely on medical facts, with no bias.

Unplanned pregnancy is common, so do remember the following:

o The morning-after Pill is effective for longer than just the day after – up to three or five days – but the earlier you take it, the better.

o There's no limit to how many times you can take the morning-after Pill.

o The copper coil can also be used as emergency contraception, but the hormone coil cannot.

o An abortion can be performed at up to twenty-four weeks of pregnancy and there are both medical and surgical options.

o Abortion does not harm your fertility in the future.

CHAPTER 9

Sexually transmitted infections

You're not just sharing germs with the person that you're having sex with; you're sharing germs with all the people that they have had sex with before you too.

I often say this to patients as a last-ditch attempt at emphasising the importance of protection against sexually transmitted infections (STIs). They are still one of the biggest taboos, as is getting tested. Every gynaecological history includes as standard the question: 'Have you ever had an STI?' to which most people will reply, 'No'. This is then followed up with: 'And when were you last tested?' to which the most common response is, 'Oh . . . I've never been tested.'

If you've never been tested then you cannot confidently say that you've never had an STI because the most common ones at least are often without symptoms, so you wouldn't necessarily know you'd had it without the test. It's also important to note that a smear test does not check for STIs; you need to go for specific tests at the sexual-health clinic, also known as the GUM (genitourinary medicine) clinic.

I remember being about fifteen years old, walking with my

dad through the hospital where he worked as a surgeon. He is very strict and old-fashioned, and in his stiffly starched white coat he was clearly identifiable as a doctor. Hence we were stopped by two men asking for directions to the GUM clinic. He turned to me and asked, 'What's the GUM clinic?' Although I didn't know what it stood for, I did know it was the sexual-health clinic, but as an embarrassed teenager I was too shy to say the word 'sexual' in front of my father. Thankfully, one of the guys said it for me, I turned a shade of beetroot and my dad gave them the directions they needed. Later, at home, I looked up the abbreviation, and to this day I've never forgotten what GUM stands for.

Many people tend to focus on contraception for preventing pregnancy yet forget about the risk of STIs. And it doesn't matter whether you're having sex with just one person at a time. If you're doing it without a condom and either of you has not been tested recently for STIs, you are at risk of either giving or receiving one. I feel very strongly about empowering women to feel it's OK to both carry and insist on using condoms. Plenty of people have told me they prefer to take the Pill because they're too embarrassed to use condoms. But, I will say it again: this does not protect you from STIs. And, arguably, women need to be the most concerned about this because they are the ones who will suffer the greatest health consequences.

Chlamydia: 'It runs in my family'

Chlamydia, the commonest STI in the UK, is a bacterial infection that shows no symptoms in about 70 per cent of infected women and 50 per cent of infected men. You can only catch it through sexual contact, so if it does 'run in the family' as a patient once informed me, it means everyone in the family should read this section to understand the importance of barrier contraception and STI screening.

The symptoms in women are vague: pain or bleeding during or after sex, bleeding in between periods, a non-specific vaginal discharge and pain when urinating. Men tend to have discharge coming from their penis, testicle pain and burning or stinging on passing urine. Shortly after I broke up with a dreadful, cheating ex-boyfriend many, many years ago, he called me and told me he had these exact symptoms and was going to get checked for chlamydia. I, of course, was terrified. Thankfully, it turned out he had a thrush infection, which, in my opinion, seemed a little less than he deserved for his misdemeanours. But it goes to show that it's hard to know what exactly is going on without the proper tests.

Due to the high rates of infection in under-twenty-fives, with about 3 per cent of the UK population being infected, an NHS national chlamydia screening programme exists, whereby sixteen- to twenty-four-year-olds are encouraged to be screened either yearly or every time they change partner. Men and women can both be tested via a urine sample, but for women a swab taken from the vagina is preferred because it is slightly more accurate.

If positive, treatment is with antibiotics – either a one-off dose, or a week-long course, which could be a tablet or injection – and you shouldn't engage in any kind of sexual activity until seven days after finishing the treatment. It's also recommended to be re-tested three months after treatment. Some studies have suggested that about 1 in 5 cases of chlamydia can clear on their own. Certainly for me, however, that rate of spontaneous clearance isn't enough to want to chance it, particularly in view of the fact that untreated chlamydia can cause pelvic inflammatory disease (see below).

A chlamydia vaccine is currently under development and

looks promising, but it will be many years before it's ready for widespread use.

Gonorrhoea

Caused by a bug called *Neisseria gonorrhoea*, it is less common than chlamydia, but the two are often found together. Gonorrhoea doesn't just cause vaginal infections, but can also infect the rectum (back passage) if you've been having anal sex, and your throat from oral sex.

I remember one case as a medical student doing my GP placement of a fifteen-year-old girl who came with a persistent throat infection that had not responded to the usual antibiotics. We took a swab and it turned out to be gonorrhoea. Because of her age and the fact that she always came in with her mother, it became quite a tricky situation because we needed to inform her sensitively, give her the appropriate antibiotics and also ensure her partners were tested and treated. Having said that, an uninfected woman is more likely to get gonorrhoea from her infected male partner, than an infected woman is to give it to her uninfected partner. Either way, everyone needs to get tested, and that's where GUM clinics can help with partner tracing, so that all the necessary people can be screened.

Urine testing is pretty ineffective for detecting gonorrhoea, so it needs to be a swab sample. Treatment is the same as for chlamydia (see pages 124–6), and since we know they like to party together, the antibiotics will cover both types of infection, treating them wherever they are in the body. Re-testing is also highly recommended due to the high rates of re-infection.

Multi-drug resistant strains of gonorrhoea are now emerging and present quite the treatment challenge, again reinforcing the need for active STI prevention.

SH:24

SH:24 is a free online sexual-health service, charity-funded and delivered in partnership with the NHS (see Resources, page 243 for details). It takes away the need for any over-the-shoulder action by delivering a sexual-health-screening kit to your door in a plain envelope. Inside, there is a swab that needs to be taken from your vagina to check for chlamydia and gonorrhoea, and a small finger-pricking device (way less scary than it sounds!), so that you can put some blood droplets into a tube to test for HIV and syphilis. You post the kit back in the envelope provided and within seven days you'll get a text message with your results. If anything comes back positive, you'll be offered the opportunity to speak to a doctor or nurse over the phone and it is likely that you will need to go to a clinic for the appropriate treatment. If that's not convenience for you, I don't know what is. Which is probably why the number of people getting tested was shown to almost double in a study that compared people who were invited to attend a clinic with those who were invited to order a home-testing kit.[60]

Trichomonas vaginalis

The textbooks and websites say this causes a 'frothy discharge'. That's not terribly helpful for you because I've seen plenty of women with *Trichomonas vaginalis* (TV), but none of them has ever told me there's a bubble bath going on down below (although upon doing a speculum examination, it is sometimes possible for the doctor or nurse to see a frothy type of discharge, and sometimes the cervix can be described as being like a strawberry in appearance because of the irritation this causes to the tissue). I love to throw this into my lectures on the cervix and ask students to give me a spot diagnosis (although a swab would still be taken to confirm). They often look at me in horror, but I'm never sure if that's because they don't know the answer or because I have turned up on many occasions to teach them en route to the gym, wearing Lululemon leggings and stilettoes. I digress. Some women report having an itchy, irritating discharge, but as with chlamydia and gonorrhoea, TV is often asymptomatic.

It is treated using metronidazole, an antibiotic tablet that you'll usually need to take for a week and your partner will also need to be tested.

Mycoplasma genitalium

Now this might be one that you've never heard of, but it's thought to infect about 1 per cent of under-forty-fives in the UK.[61] As with the previously mentioned infections, it causes pretty ambiguous symptoms, including abnormal vaginal discharge, pain on urinating and bleeding after sex or between periods. Again, it's detected most effectively using a vaginal swab rather than a urine test and is treated with antibiotics. It can cause long-term health complications including pelvic inflammatory disease (see pages 130–1) and premature delivery if present in pregnancy.[62]

Syphilis

Previously the disease of kings, artists and dictators, many people think this one has died out, but in fact it's coming back with a vengeance in the UK, with levels currently higher than they've been since 1949. It's caused by a bacterium *Treponema pallidum*, and left untreated, it can cause very severe health problems.

Ulcers/sores will appear on your genitals, mouth or anus about two to three weeks after contracting the infection. They're not normally painful and can leak a clear fluid, which is like a highly infectious soup containing the bugs. They'll disappear about six weeks later, but this doesn't mean the infection has gone. A secondary outbreak can occur with very non-specific symptoms, including rashes, fatigue and joint pains, and these may come and go. Over years and decades, the infection can ultimately spread to your brain and heart and also cause non-cancerous tumour growth in various locations. However, it is totally preventable through screening and treatment.

Syphilis is diagnosed with a blood, unless the active ulcers are present, in which case a swab can be taken from the fluid coming from them. Antibiotics, often as an injection, are effective at treating syphilis.

We routinely screen pregnant women during the first antenatal appointment and I've seen a surprising number diagnosed at this point who were never aware that they had the infection. One particularly distraught patient asked me how it was possible since she had only ever had one sexual partner. I think the idea that you need to be sexually adventurous or promiscuous to get an STI is one of the reasons that we don't always prioritise screening – yet it is the only way to prevent their spread. Syphilis in pregnancy can spread to the baby via the placenta and may require treatment and extra scans due to the high risk of congenital abnormalities, as well as miscarriage and premature delivery.[63]

Pelvic Inflammatory Disease (PID)

STIs and other non-sexually transmitted bacteria, such as the type that cause bacterial vaginosis and also those from your bowel, can cause inflammation of the upper female reproductive tract – the endometrium (uterine lining), fallopian tubes, ovaries and pelvic cavity – due to the upward spread of infections in the vagina and cervix, which can be facilitated by having sex, the backward flow of menstrual blood and also having a coil inserted.

Chlamydia, gonorrhoea and, to a lesser extent, *Mycoplasma genitalium* are the usual suspects[64] and it's important to stress that even when you don't have any symptoms with these infections, they can still be getting up to no good and causing damage inside.

Acute PID can start about six weeks after initial infection, causing often quite severe lower-abdominal pain, abnormal vaginal discharge, bleeding after sex and in between periods, pain during sex and fevers. It can sometimes require admission to hospital, and the common theme is usually 'But I've never had an STI . . . ' But they've also usually never been tested. I don't blame the patients; I blame a lack of education about the importance of STI testing.

Treatment is a two-week course of antibiotics. Untreated acute PID can lead to chronic PID, where the ongoing inflammation leads to the formation of scar tissue that can cause your womb and bowel to stick together and to the pelvic side-walls, resulting in chronic pelvic pain. This can also cause infertility by blocking the fallopian tubes and therefore STI screening is always one of the first things we do to investigate if a woman cannot get pregnant. Adhesions in the pelvic cavity can be broken down during keyhole surgery and chlamydia infection has a very classic cobweb appearance that we see as soon as we start the operation. Scarring inside the fallopian tubes themselves is not removable, so IVF may eventually be needed to get pregnant. There is also a higher risk of ectopic pregnancy, because while the tube may not be completely blocked, it's too small for a growing fertilised egg to travel through, so it gets stuck.

This might all sound a bit scary and dramatic, but it's a pertinent reminder of why we can't be blasé about the need to prevent, screen and treat STIs.

Genital warts

There's a lot of confusion about genital warts and herpes. Warts are caused by the human papilloma virus (HPV) that can also cause cervical cancer (see Chapter 10), although it's the 'low-risk' types that cause warts, not to be confused with the 'high-risk' types that cause cervical cancer. Having warts doesn't automatically put you at a higher risk of cervical cancer.

HPV warts are pink and fleshy, and can be itchy, but don't often cause a lot of problems and you may just feel some little lumps. It can take up to eighteen months from infection for the warts to show, so it can be incredibly difficult to work out where you got it from, which often causes a lot of distress – plus, we always want someone to blame. Such is the taboo around warts that several patients have insisted the lab must be wrong when I've removed them and the result states 'HPV wart'. But the virus is everywhere, and it's really easy to contract via skin-to-skin contact, so condoms are the only way to reduce the risk of infection but it's very difficult to prevent completely. Partners will only need treatment if they have warts themselves.

The current HPV vaccine protects against the two most

common wart-forming types of HPV: HPV-6 and -11. In Australia, where the vaccine has been very well publicised, HPV warts have almost died out.[65] I hope the same will be seen in the UK if we can increase the number of people having the vaccine.

Most warts will disappear on their own within two years, but they can, if desired, be treated with various liquids and pastes, or also be frozen off, usually at a sexual-health clinic.

Herpes

Genital herpes is caused by the herpes simplex virus (HSV) types 1 and 2, which also cause cold sores.

I once reviewed a young girl in A&E with her first episode of genital herpes. She told me she hadn't had sex for over two years. I asked her whether she'd had oral sex recently. She seemed slightly shocked to be asked this by a doctor, but she nodded. What many people don't realise is that most women can get genital herpes from receiving oral sex from someone with a cold sore – which is ironic because cold sores don't carry the horrible stigma that genital herpes does. The virus cannot travel from a cold sore to your own genitals though, unless you happen to be a body contortionist. It occurs through direct skin-to-skin contact, entering the body through tiny tears in the tissue and travelling along sensory nerves, which is why the blisters can be so painful. I always feel terribly sorry for women who often can't even wee without experiencing excruciating pain, so I usually give them some local anaesthetic gel to use on the area.

The risk of transmission is highest when the blisters are present, but it is also possible when they're not.[66] The blisters will crust over and disappear within four weeks following the first outbreak and within about twelve days in recurrent episodes.[67] Antiviral medication – available only on prescription – can be used to shorten the duration of a herpes outbreak and can even prevent recurrence entirely if taken early enough. Aciclovir cream for cold sores is available over the counter and can be used on genital herpes, but is not as effective as the tablets.[67]

A blood test can tell if you've had the infection before, but not where you had it (i.e. a cold sore or genital herpes) or for how long. Genital herpes can only be diagnosed by a swab from a sore.

Some women may require treatment from thirty-six weeks of pregnancy onwards to reduce the risk of transmitting the infection to their baby during a vaginal delivery. This will be discussed with your obstetrician in antenatal clinic.

Human immunodeficiency virus (HIV)

HIV is a virus that destroys white blood cells, which are a necessary part of a healthy immune system. AIDS stands for acquired immunodeficiency syndrome and refers to a large collection of infections and complications that can result from being infected by HIV. HIV and AIDS are not the same thing, and not everyone with HIV will get AIDS, especially if treated early.

HIV has generally been regarded as a disease of gay men, but this is very much not the case, with almost half of all new cases diagnosed in the UK each year being in heterosexual men and women.[68] I admit that I myself was initially shocked when I saw young women being diagnosed with the virus. They were your average twenty-something girls, went to university, had jobs, a few boyfriends, but not more than one at a time. Why were they getting HIV? Because they didn't think they'd be at risk and were not using barrier contraception.

Anyone having unprotected sex is at risk of getting the virus. Yes, the risk is very low compared to other STIs, but it's not zero, and that's a message that we really need to get out there.

HIV can also be caught through sharing needles – and not just for drugs; think backstreet tattoo parlours or even a cut-price Botox party. Any kind of needle is single-use. End of.

HIV is diagnosed by a blood test, which is also part of the routine antenatal screening for pregnant women (because the virus can be passed via the placenta to the unborn child, and during delivery).

Antiviral medication (prescription only) is highly effective for HIV, and although it can't completely cure the infection, it has been shown to result in near-normal life expectancy.[69] If the treatment manages to drop the viral load (a measure of how much virus is in the body) to 'undetectable', the infection cannot then be passed on.[70]

|||||||||||||||||||||||||||||||||||||||||||

THINGS YOU'VE ALWAYS WANTED TO KNOW, BUT WERE TOO AFRAID TO ASK

When do I need to get checked for STIs?
You need to be checked for STIs:

- if you have symptoms
- if you are starting a new relationship and planning on having sex without a condom
- if you have had sex without a condom and don't know whether your partner had any infections.

Also, bear in mind the amount of time it takes for particular infections to reliably show up on the tests: for chlamydia and gonorrhoea, it's two weeks; for HIV, four weeks; for syphilis, three months.

How do I take a self-sample swab for STI testing?

It's really simple to take a self-sample vaginal swab for STI testing, and it can even be taken when you're having your period or having spotting. It won't affect the results.

You may wish to sit on the toilet while you take the swab or stand with one foot up on the top of the toilet.

Step 1 Wash your hands.
Step 2 Insert the swab tip about 5cm up into your vagina.
Step 3 Twist the swab around for fifteen to thirty seconds, so that it touches the walls of your vagina.
Step 4 Remove the swab and put it straight into the tube it came in and close it firmly.
Step 5 Relax and feel very proud of yourself!

Can I get an STI from oral sex?

While you can't get pregnant through oral sex, there's no 'safe route' when it comes to infections. This is because the tissue in your mouth and throat (and also around your rectum) is very similar to that in your vagina, or inside a penis, so any of the bugs that can infect your genitals can also infect your mouth – they're not fussy, they just want a moist, warm home. Gonorrhoea, herpes and HPV are most likely to infect the oral cavity. Chlamydia, syphilis and HIV can all also be transmitted via oral sex, although the chances are lower.[71]

Commonly available antiseptic mouthwashes are being investigated as a potential way of reducing the risk of oral gonorrhoea transmission, and have shown promising results.[72,73]

However, the only certain way to prevent oral transmission of STIs if you're not sure that both you and your partner are negative is to use condoms or a dental dam. I know, you're probably thinking, a dental whaaaaat? Well, it's a flat sheet that is placed over your vulva during oral sex. I've searched high and low for them in a variety of outlets in London, from pharmacies to high-street sex shops, but have only ever managed to find them online. (It's all in the name of market research!) The moral of the story? Get tested to stay safe.

||||||||||||||||||||||||||||||||||||||||||||

THE GYNAE GEEK'S KNOWLEDGE BOMBS

I used to work in a gynaecology department in central London that was across the road from a very large sexual-health clinic. Pretty much everyone who went there would give a cursory glance over their shoulder and then walk in with a guilty look on their face, head hanging slightly in shame. I always wanted to high-five them for having the nerve to go, but I thought that might put them off even more!

We need to normalise the idea of going to the sexual-health clinic to remove the stigma. With this in mind, please remember these key points:

- If you've never been tested for STIs you cannot confidently say you've never had one. There is nothing shameful about going to a sexual-health clinic, it's a sign of being a responsible adult.
- Anyone can have an STI, regardless of how many people they've had sex with and whether they look clean or smell nice.
- Online self-testing kits are available if you're too embarrassed to go to a clinic. There are no excuses!
- Chlamydia is the most common bacterial STI and causes no symptoms in about 70 per cent of infected women.
- You can still get STIs from oral and anal sex.

CHAPTER 10

Cervical screening and HPV vaccination

'I've never had a smear test because it sounds too painful.'

Every time I hear this, I die a little inside. Having said that, I must have far more than nine lives because I hear it on such a frequent basis. Cervical screening (or 'smear testing') is the single best way of reducing your risk of a cervical cancer, which, in the UK, has a lifetime risk of 1 in 135.[22]

Contrary to popular belief, cervical screening is not a cervical cancer test, but is aimed at picking up abnormal cells before they turn into cancer, so that they can be treated to reduce the risk of them doing so in the future. I see countless women who don't understand what a smear test is for, which I is why, I think, so many don't have them; and I also see women in the colposcopy clinic (where you are investigated if you have an abnormal smear) who are absolutely distraught, convinced that they have cancer because they don't understand what their test results mean.

Cervical cancer and HPV

Cervical cancer is caused by the human papilloma virus (HPV), of which there are hundreds of types, at least fifteen of which, called 'high-risk HPV', are known to cause cervical cancer, as well as cancers of the vagina, vulva, throat, anus and penis. Other types can cause genital warts (see Chapter 9).

I always describe HPV to my patients as 'the common cold that you get on your cervix. Pretty much everyone gets it, and most people clear it quickly. And if you don't clear it, you start to get changes in the cells, which is what we are trying to pick up in your smear test.'

By the age of fifty, at least 90 per cent of women will have been infected with a high-risk HPV, but 0.75 per cent get cervical cancer – so something isn't really adding up here, is it? And that's because the immune system clears the infection in most women. In some people, this happens incredibly quickly – possibly within a few days – but in others, it can take weeks, months or even years. If it hangs about, it starts to cause changes in the cells because the virus is a bit needy and has to make a comfy home in your ever-so-hospitable cervical cells to help it survive. It's these cellular changes that we are looking for in a smear test. Think of it as a bit of a housing inspection: are you sub-letting your cervix to HPV?

The cellular changes are called cervical intraepithelial neoplasia (CIN) and are 'precancerous' – because if the HPV remains, they can become more abnormal and eventually turn into cervical cancer. From first infection, however, this usually takes at least ten to fifteen years. During this time, you will have been invited for between three and five cervical smears through which we can detect the abnormal cells and treat you before they ever turn into cancer. This means that attending your smear tests is the single most effective way of preventing cervical cancer.

Most people think they've never had HPV because they have never had an abnormal smear test. But HPV is all over the place. It is in our environment and all over our skin. In fact, a study has even found high-risk HPV on the hands of small children.[74] Chances are, if you've ever been sexually active, you've probably had the virus on your cervix because that's how it gets there. You just don't know about it because your body cleared it quickly, and you didn't happen to have a smear during the time that HPV was setting up shop in your cervix.

Finding out you have HPV doesn't mean your partner is cheating on you. I like to think I've kept a lot of relationships together, given the number of times I've had women crying in my clinic, saying they are going to break up with their boyfriend or husband because they've obviously been cheating. Their partner may well have given them the virus, I explain, but that doesn't mean they've been cheating at all. As I said, the virus is everywhere, so even being in an exclusive relationship with one person for the rest of your life can't prevent you from getting it. That's also the reason why condoms won't always protect you from HPV like they will other STIs. 'I've never had sex with a man, so I don't need a smear test' is a common misconception because having a same-sex partner won't protect you either. We've all heard of 'boy germs' . . . well, HPV isn't one of them. It's on men and women and it's everywhere, so if you've ever performed any kind of sexual act that has involved inserting anything into your vagina, by yourself, a man or a woman, you still need to get tested because the virus is everywhere. And that's why everyone who has ever had sex needs to go for smear tests to check for potentially precancerous changes, so they can be treated to prevent a cancer in the long term.

Smear tests

Hopefully, by now, I've managed to convince you that smear tests are important enough for you to want to get one. So how do you go about it?

You'll get a letter inviting you for a smear test shortly before your twenty-fifth birthday, then every three years from then on, and every five years after the age of fifty. I wouldn't recommend anyone to have a smear test more often than that because there is a risk of over-detecting mild, insignificant disease that will go away of its own accord, which unnecessarily increases anxiety and can lead to over-treatment, which has its risks (see pages 150–151).

What happens?

There isn't really an 'ideal' time of your menstrual cycle to go for a smear test,[75] although it's best avoided during your period.

You'll be asked to lie down and the person taking the smear will explain how to position your legs. A plastic speculum is then inserted, which can be a bit uncomfortable when it's opened up to find your cervix, but after that, it takes just a few seconds to collect the sample using a soft plastic brush.

The results will take a few weeks and if it's abnormal, you'll be automatically referred to the colposcopy department at your nearest hospital.

It's very common to get some spotting after the smear test, especially if you have an ectropion (see pages 11–13), which is not a sign of anything untoward or that the doctor/nurse did something wrong; it's simply that the brush scratched your cervix and made it bleed. A lot of women have cried after they've seen me removing a slightly blood-stained brush after taking their smear, thinking it's a sign that something is wrong. However, this kind of bleeding or an ectropion do not increase your chance of having abnormalities or of getting cancer. You might also feel a bit of period-like pain, again from stimulation of the cervix. It will go in a few hours, but it's OK to take paracetamol and ibuprofen if you want. A tilted uterus (see pages 16–17) can also make it slightly more uncomfortable, but only for a few seconds.

A small number of people can feel quite faint after having a smear because touching the cervix with the brush can reduce your blood pressure. Please don't feel embarrassed to say you feel unwell, as it's easier for us to help you lie down and give you some water, than it is to scrape you off the floor when you've hit the deck and maybe hurt yourself in the process.

Abnormal results

In the UK, about 95 per cent of women attending cervical screening will have a normal result. They don't need to do anything further and will automatically get another letter to go for a test a few years later.

For the 1 in 20 who have an abnormal result it can be a very worrying and confusing time. But an abnormal result does not mean that you have cervical cancer. It means that the screening suggests you may have abnormal cells on your cervix that need to be looked at more closely because you may have a precancerous abnormality (CIN). It's a slow-growing disease, so it's not possible for it to change into a cancer between having the smear and going to your colposcopy appointment.

Here are the abnormal results you could get, how common they are and what they broadly correspond to...

Borderline changes	2%	HPV-related changes in the cells, no CIN present.	Likely to go away without treatment
Low-grade/mild dyskaryosis	2%	CIN1	
High-grade/ moderate dyskaryosis	0.5%	CIN2	Likely to need treatment (see below)
High-grade/severe dyskaryosis	0.6%	CIN3	
High-grade dyskaryosis ? invasion	0.01%	Possibly cervical cancer, although many will turn out to be only CIN3	

Dyskaryosis is a long, difficult-to-pronounce way of saying abnormal-looking cells. Borderline and low-grade changes are only referred to colposcopy if there is high-risk HPV present – because if there isn't, you don't have the driver present (HPV) to continue their abnormal growth into a cancer. It may be that you did have high-risk HPV and it's gone and the cells are on their way back to normal, or you have a low-risk HPV which will never turn the cells into a cancer.

A small number of women may get a result stating 'inadequate'; this simply means there were not enough cells in the sample to get an accurate result. This does not increase the risk of actually having an underlying abnormality, but means you'll need the test repeating in three months. It's also more common after the menopause.

Colposcopy

Pronounced 'kol-POS-kuh-pee'. Definition: 1. Using a microscope to look at your colpos; Greek for womb 2. A word to terrify and alarm women far and wide.

It's completely normal to be scared on your first visit, and lots of women walk in and start crying immediately, which often helps me know who might need a bit more reassurance. I always ask at the end, 'Was it as bad as you were expecting?' to which 99 per cent say, 'No'. About 25 per cent also hug me – but don't feel obliged!

So why do we offer this scary-sounding examination? So that we can look directly at your cervix, to see if you really do have any abnormal cells, as the screening is not completely accurate and often overcalls the result. About 40 per cent of women going for a colposcopy will actually have a completely normal cervix at the time of examination.

Some people may also need to come for a colposcopy without an abnormal smear test. This would include someone with bleeding after sex or between periods, or who had an examination by someone else (say, at the sexual-health clinic) who thought their cervix didn't look quite normal.

What happens?

To start with, it's quite similar to a smear test. You'll lie down on the couch with the stirrups to support your legs (these can be offputting for a lot of people, but it means you're in a better position for us to find your cervix). After the speculum is inserted we'll have a good look at your cervix (and as hard as we look, we can't see your ovaries, as many women will ask – see Chapter 2 if you're wondering why). We put some liquids on the cervix using cotton wool. The first is acetic acid, which smells like vinegar and the second is iodine, which you may remember from science at school as being a dark brown solution. I'm known for being messy and sloshing things around during a colposcopy, as a result of which my favourite black heels have a big brown stain on their pale beige lining from where I dripped iodine all over them – whoops! You will be given a gown to wear, so that we don't ruin your clothes.

If there are any abnormal areas, we may take some biopsies. These are tiny pieces of tissue that we can send to the lab to get a more accurate diagnosis. Having a biopsy taken isn't necessarily a worrying sign, as many patients feel. In fact, there is a small amount of evidence to suggest that taking a biopsy can actually stimulate an immune reaction to kickstart clearance of HPV infection and abnormal cells.[76]

Treatment for abnormal cells

Mild abnormalities (CIN1) are not usually treated because the majority go back to normal on their own over time, so we prefer to watch and wait. Patients often ask why we can't just remove the cells, so that they don't have to worry and keep coming back. This isn't recommended, however, because treatment can slightly increase the risk of late miscarriage and premature birth in future pregnancies. It's important to note that treatment does not affect fertility though, which is something my colleagues and I researched during my Ph.D.,[77] in response to the number of patients who asked about this in clinic.

More severe abnormalities (CIN 2 and 3) are usually treated because they have a higher risk of turning into a cancer in the future, over years, maybe even decades. Not all cases will do so, but, because we cannot predict who this will happen to, we currently recommend treatment in most cases. This may involve excision (cutting out the abnormal cells) or ablation (burning them off or destroying them). Most treatment for CIN in the UK is performed using excision, often known as a LLETZ, which stands for:

Large – don't let this worry you; it's only going to be as big as it needs to be to remove all the abnormal cells, which, in some cases, is quite small

Loop – loop of wire

Excision – cutting away of the

Transformation **Z**one – the name for the specific area of the cervix where CIN develops

What happens?

Treatment can be done in the outpatient clinic with local anaesthetic. You'll need to eat and drink as normal on the day, as I've had a lot of women fainting on me afterwards because of hypoglycaemia. In our clinic we have an impressive chocolate stash, so if you do faint, you'll probably wake up with me standing over you and simultaneously fanning you, while shoving a chocolate button under your lip.

Drama aside, it's generally pretty quick, simple and my patients are usually pleasantly surprised. Some small local anaesthetic injections are given, and judging by most patients' reactions, this isn't as painful as it sounds. 'Oh . . . you've already done it?' many women say, although the fact that I am usually chatting for England probably helps. Of course, not everyone treats a colposcopy appointment like a coffee morning, so if your colposcopist isn't chatty, they're probably just concentrating (and that's not a bad thing), but there will be a nurse there to distract you and talk to you throughout.

A small loop of wire with an electric current going through is used to remove the cells, which usually takes a minute or two. Afterwards, a small ball on a stick may be used to stop any bleeding, or a brown paste applied called Monsel's solution.

It's a good idea to take someone with you to the appointment in case you don't feel great afterwards. They don't have to go in with you, but it's nice to have someone to go and get a cup of tea with afterwards, before slowly making your way home. That said, I've had some women who dash in, I cut out their CIN and they're hotfooting it straight down to Oxford Street to take advantage of the fact they have the afternoon off work! Everyone is different.

Aftercare – Glastonbury Festival is still OK

If there's ever an excuse for a duvet day, having a cervical treatment has to be one of them. Go home afterwards, change into something comfy and do something to completely relax.

You shouldn't use tampons/menstrual cups, swim or have sex for the next two to four weeks, in order to give the cervix time to heal without the risk of introducing infections. When the bleeding/discharge has stopped, you're good to go with all of the above if you feel ready. Regarding exercise, some doctors advise against it for the same period of time in case it disturbs the healing scab. However, in reality, plenty of women continue to exercise with no problem at all, having taken it easy for the first few days, just to give the scab time to form properly. You know your body best; listen to it and do as you see fit.

By way of illustration, I was once at Glastonbury Festival when one of my friends came up to me and said that the scab had just fallen off her cervix, following an LLETZ she'd had a few weeks earlier. It was probably ready to fall off anyway, so even the most energetic dancing at the Pyramid Stage was unlikely to have properly dislodged it. So what I'm trying to say is, be prepared to take it easy for a few weeks, but you don't have to put your life on hold.

You will need a repeat smear and HPV test at six months. If you get pregnant in the future you should make sure you tell your midwife at your booking appointment that you've had a treatment before, because you may need extra scans of your cervix, depending on how much tissue you had removed and how long your cervix is early on in the pregnancy.

HPV vaccine

Natural infection does offer some protection, but it is much, much less than that offered by the recently developed HPV vaccines. They can protect against HPV for over a decade at least, and with more and more evidence emerging, we know it will ultimately give protection for a lot longer. We just haven't had it long enough to prove this.

The currently used vaccine protects against HPV-16 and HPV-18 which cause about 70 per cent of cervical cancers, and also HPV-6 and HPV-11 which cause genital warts. A new vaccine coming out in the next few years will include protection against more types of cancer-causing HPV and could therefore prevent up to 90 per cent of cervical cancer.[78]

A lot of parents feel uncomfortable about vaccinating young girls against a virus that is related to sex, and while I don't think anyone really knows the right time to discuss sex with a child, it has been well proven that the vaccine is far more effective when given before there has been natural exposure to the virus, and therefore before having sex for the first time. In the UK, the vaccine is given at twelve to thirteen years, with a second dose given six months later.

The first cohort of vaccinated girls are now at the age at which they're starting cervical screening and I have had several coming to clinic with abnormalities. Most of them were vaccinated when they were older than twelve to thirteen and had had sex prior to vaccination. This means they haven't got as much benefit from the vaccine as they would if it had been given before they started having sex. It's also important to remember it doesn't protect against every type of HPV, so you still need to be screened after being vaccinated.

Is the vaccine safe?

The anti-vax gang have a much stronger publicity campaign than the healthcare providers and governments who want to vaccinate their patients and populations, yet a far weaker evidence base. There are some case reports of girls getting chronic fatigue syndrome and POTS (postural orthostatic tachycardia syndrome – a condition that causes abnormal increases in heart rate when sitting or standing) after vaccination. However, the numbers are tiny compared to the millions of women that have been vaccinated, and hence protected against cervical cancer, with numerous large studies failing to show any association between the vaccine and the aforementioned conditions.[79,80] So even if these cases are a result of the vaccine, they are *incredibly* rare. We must remember that no medical treatment is without risk, and so we have to weigh things up.

Note: it does not contain a live virus, so you absolutely cannot get HPV or any HPV-related cancer from having the jab.

The common side effects of the vaccine are similar to those of most others and include feeling a bit under the weather as your immune system is kicking into action and that oh-so-delightful 'dead-arm' feeling, with a bit of redness at the injection site, all of which will disappear within twenty-four to forty-eight hours.

What about the boys?

Ideally, we should vaccinate boys – not only to protect women, but also to reduce their risk of HPV-related cancers such as throat, anal and penile cancers and, of course, genital warts as well. Unfortunately, it's not available on the NHS at the moment. However, the current evidence has shown that by vaccinating girls we do still get pretty good 'herd immunity'; that means the boys get protection from the girls being vaccinated.[81] If you want to get your son vaccinated, you can do this through a private healthcare provider, and I know several mothers who have done so. As with women, it will have a better effect if it's done at a young age, prior to starting sexual activity.

IIIIIIIIIIIIIIIIIIIIIIIIIIIIIIIIIIIIII

THINGS YOU'VE ALWAYS WANTED TO KNOW, BUT WERE TOO AFRAID TO ASK

Why can't I get a smear test before the age of twenty-five?

Screening from a younger age does not reduce the risk of cervical cancer, which has been shown in other countries where it is done. HPV infection rates and mild abnormalities are common in women under twenty-five, and the younger you are, the more likely the infection will clear and the cells to go back to normal, which is why cervical cancer is exceedingly rare under twenty-five.

To prevent one case of cervical cancer in the twenty-to-twenty-four age group requires screening up to 40,000 women and treating up to 900.[82] This is because we know most changes go back to normal on their own. As someone who runs colposcopy clinics where we see women with abnormal smears, I can tell you that's a lot of very scared women who need to come to clinic for no benefit, and involves treating a lot of women in whom it won't even prevent cancer, while putting them at a higher risk of pregnancy complications.

Medicine is a minefield of risks and benefits. There are, of course, women who are unfortunately diagnosed with cervical cancer below the age of twenty-five, and it's difficult to work out how this can be prevented. A lot of these cases also tend to be unusual types of cancer that would not be picked up by screening which, in any case, can never prevent 100 per cent of cases. So please go for your test when you're invited. It's the best twenty-fifth birthday present you could hope for!

I've never had sex before. Do I need a smear?

Given that HPV is spread through genital contact you are unlikely to ever get cervical cancer if you've never been sexually active, so you do not absolutely need to attend screening. But if you've ever had intercourse or genital contact, even just once, you still need to go.

I went to my GP with abnormal vaginal bleeding, but they wouldn't do a smear test – why?

Where can I find your GP to give them a pat on the back?

This is entirely correct. A smear test is a screening test. That means it's designed to pick out people from a population who are high risk for having a disease (in this case CIN), but do not have symptoms. Abnormal vaginal bleeding, e.g. in between periods or after sex, is a symptom and may represent an underlying disease. That means you need a diagnostic test, such as an ultrasound or a colposcopy to further investigate your symptoms.

I've had CIN treated before. Should I have the vaccine?

Given that you're at a slightly higher risk of getting CIN in the future it has been suggested it may be particularly beneficial,[83] but more evidence is needed before it can become routine practice. If you want it, you would have to pay to have it done privately. While it won't do any harm, you can't expect the same degree of protection it would give to a child because you've been exposed to HPV before. The same is true for other adults who want to get the vaccine and haven't had treatment before.

Is there a natural way to get rid of HPV?

There is no medication to treat HPV. Although a lot of patients tell me they've been to herbal doctors who have given them mysterious concoctions that have cleared HPV, none of this is evidence-based. There are, however, several studies suggesting that consumption of a diet rich in fruit and vegetables may increase the chances of clearing the infection.[84]

|||||||||||||||||||||||||||||||||||||||||||||

THE GYNAE GEEK'S KNOWLEDGE BOMBS

HPV infection is very common and sounds really scary. But it doesn't have to be. Unfortunately, you can't do anything to stop yourself getting the infection, but smear testing is the single best way to prevent yourself getting cervical cancer. Remember these points to stay informed:

- HPV infection is not a sign of promiscuity. It's everywhere, but sex gets it to your cervix.
- Smear tests don't check for STIs, for any other cancers or tell you anything about your fertility.
- Testing more often, or from a younger age doesn't make you any less likely to get cervical cancer.
- Treatment for abnormal cells is simple, but is only done in cases of severe precancer; milder cases will go away on their own and treatment may increase the risk of problems in a future pregnancy.

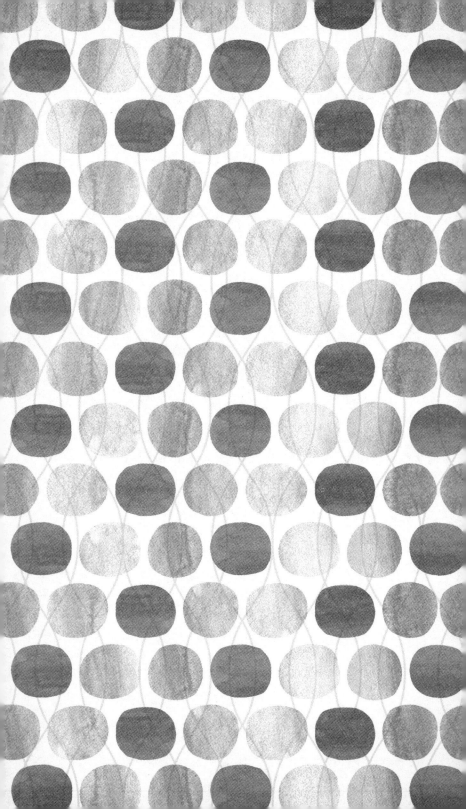

PART FOUR

Fertility and Getting Pregnant

Some of you may already have children. I'm assuming the rest of you fall into one of three categories:

- You're thinking about having a baby in the short/medium term.
- You haven't really thought about it, but you might consider it in the future
- It's totally not on your radar.

But it doesn't matter which category you're in. It's important to be more aware of your fertility, which isn't something we think that much about until we want to use it to have a baby.

Fifty per cent of pregnancies are planned, and many of those are done so meticulously. But does it need to be like that? And what about fertility tests? Supplements? There's very little reliable information about this online, and a lot of it seems to exist in chatrooms and forums. This section will cover that period between making the decision to try for a baby, to the point where you need to pee on a stick.

I'll also cover egg freezing, which seems to have received a lot of coverage lately, especially since many Silicon Valley companies have started offering it to their employees. Women are intrigued, but it's quite an involved process that requires a lot of decisions to be made before doing it. And it's not something you can just pop out and do during your lunch break.

So read on for the fertility-related info that every woman should know, regardless of where 'Having a baby' sits on her to-do list.

CHAPTER 11

When you are thinking about trying to conceive

Patient: *Doctor, I'm thinking about trying to get pregnant. What do I need to do?*

Me: *Errr . . . have unprotected sex on a frequent basis.*

Patient: *Well, yes, obviously. But which tests should I do beforehand to make sure everything's OK?*

Getting pregnant has become more and more medicalised over the last few years. Many of us spend our late teens, twenties and even thirties desperately trying not to get pregnant. Then, when it comes to using our fertility, we're terrified.

Eighty-four per cent of couples will get pregnant within one year of having regular, unprotected sex. That means that one in seven couples will struggle to get pregnant. This is something that a good friend mentioned in his speech at his wedding. The audience were visibly shocked, which was interesting, given a large number were also doctors, yet I found it quite refreshing to hear someone mention a hugely taboo subject so openly. But if something actually happens to the minority of people why are we so scared? And I don't think the number of 'fertility checks' being offered online and in private clinics helps the situation. Why do we need to investigate something that isn't a problem for most? Largely, because it's big business. For the vast majority of women, it isn't necessary and probably increases anxiety.

If you've read Chapter 3, you should have a better idea of how your menstrual cycle works, which is arguably the most valuable information you can be armed with when starting to try for a pregnancy. There are also a few other things that can be done to optimise the oven that you want to put the proverbial bun into. So read on for the non-commercially driven intel on getting pregnant.

Stopping contraception

With the exception of the contraceptive injection, there is no delay in a return to fertility with any kind of hormonal contraception.[1-3] Coming off the Pill will result in your usual bleed, which generally lasts no longer than normal. However, don't panic if you typically begin a new pack of pills before the bleeding has finished. It's not really the act of taking the pills again that stops the bleeding. Many people go straight back to having a regular cycle, but for others it might take a few months to settle back into a pattern. If your period doesn't appear, go back to Chapter 7 to consider some of the possible reasons, and see your GP if it hasn't come back within six months. The same applies to the hormonal coil.

The contraceptive injection may result in up to a two-year delay in the return of fertility in extreme cases,[4] so if you are looking at getting pregnant in the near future, it is worth switching to something else in the lead-up.

Fertility check-up: a worthwhile investment?

The common fertility checks offered commercially by private clinics are hormone tests and ultrasound scans. You can't do any fertility checks on the NHS unless you haven't managed to get pregnant after a year. And many people feel that isn't fair – that they should be able to find out about their fertility if they want to. But it's not just about money here. If you do tests that aren't medically warranted, you can often find slight abnormalities ('incidental findings') that have no influence on your health or, in this case, whether you get pregnant, and which just add to anxiety.

Hormone tests usually include oestrogen, progesterone, LH and FSH. The principle is to check you're ovulating. Anti-Mullerian hormone (AMH) is another commonly offered test. This test was originally created for use in women undergoing IVF, but while it is able to give you an estimation of how many eggs you've got left in your ovaries (the higher the value the better), it doesn't accurately predict how likely you are to get pregnant.[5] AMH can be deceptively lower while you're taking the Pill[6] and women with PCOS will have quite high values,[7] so do bear that in mind if you do the test, because it may falsely reassure or alarm you. That's why tests should always be ordered by someone who is qualified in interpreting the results. You can also have an ultrasound to check 'antral follicle count', which is another way of estimating egg stocks but also doesn't accurately predict your chance of a pregnancy. Both the scan and the blood test were designed for women undergoing IVF, so they're not always applicable to a natural pregnancy.

I might check 'just for fun'

As I tell all my patients, friends, friends of friends, friends of friends of friends (i.e. pretty much most women I've ever met) – ultimately, it's up to you if you want to pay to have these tests. But there are a few things to consider:

If you go fishing for problems, you might find them, but

they are unlikely to be relevant if you're in the six out of seven couples who get pregnant with no trouble.

How will it change your management? This is something that is drummed into us at medical school. Essentially, don't do a test if the result won't make you do anything different. In this case that means if you found out you have a low number of eggs, would it prompt you to start trying to get pregnant? Would you sign up to every dating app going in the hope of finding the father of your children? Or would it go the other way? A friend left me a tearful voicemail a few years ago, telling me she had checked her AMH 'just for fun' and it was low. I was in the middle of a set of night shifts and I forgot to call her back. A few weeks later she called me again and I answered, full of apologies, but she interrupted me and said, 'Ummmm . . . Anita . . . I've actually just had a positive pregnancy test.' She had become lax with contraception and, in so doing, had demonstrated how useless AMH can be for predicting fertility.

Random sex or organised fun?

It's advised to have regular, unprotected sex two or three times a week when trying to get pregnant. Of course, with our busy lives and couples often spending days, weeks and even months apart on a regular basis that can be tricky. You're fertile for five days before you release an egg and the twenty-four hours after. It's been suggested that your greatest chance of success is actually two days before ovulation.[8] With this in mind, a lot of couples want to use the timed-intercourse principle. This means concentrating on having sex during this fertile period – therefore less sex in exchange for a higher chance of pregnancy. However, unless you're using very sophisticated techniques, it's not always that easy to predict when you ovulate. For that reason, many studies have actually shown timed intercourse generally doesn't increase your chances of pregnancy when compared to haphazard sex.[9]

'Come on, Doc – I don't have time for that much sex'

OK, OK. So there are some ways that you can try and increase your chances with timed intercourse, based on improving how accurately you predict ovulation. Ovulation tests are urine strips that can give you an idea of whether you may have released an egg. LH is a hormone released by the brain which causes ovulation, and you get a massive surge of it just prior to the release of an egg – so the test doesn't actually detect that an egg was released, but tells you you've made a decent amount of LH. This might be helpful if you're trying to get to know your cycle, but arguably, you can do the same thing by looking out for the ovulation discharge that I mentioned earlier (see pages 75–6). Your temperature will also go up slightly at ovulation (about 0.3°C), which you can also look out for by taking your temperature every morning.

With PCOS, it's a bit tricky to use these techniques to track ovulation. The reason is that you often get several spikes in LH per month because your body is desperately trying to release an egg, and ovulation strips can be positive for several days. This can make ovulation tests and even temperature monitoring slightly unreliable.

Male fertility: it takes two to tango

Men are lucky. Or are they? They don't have a fertile window; they always have swimmers ready and waiting to go and their fertility is affected much less dramatically by age. But men still have hormones that control sperm production – and they don't have periods to alert them that something could be amiss. From speaking to couples in fertility clinic, men often seem surprised at the suggestion that their fertility could be the cause of why their partner is not getting pregnant.

In fact, at least 30 per cent of fertility-related problems are due to male factors, and sperm count has halved since the 1970s, according to a study involving 43,000 men worldwide.[10] Smoking is known to affect sperm count and quality,[11] as is heavy drinking.[12] Male body weight also has a significant impact on fertility,[13] so if you're trying to improve your dietary and exercise habits, it's worth getting your partner involved too, so that you have a higher chance of sticking to it, and optimise health for both of you.

Food for fertility – more than just oysters?

Me: *Would you say you have a healthy diet?*

Couple being investigated for infertility:
Not really. We don't eat a lot of fruit or veg. And we get takeaway a few times a week. But that's OK, isn't it?'

A recently published study showed that women eating fast food on a frequent basis took longer to fall pregnant, and those who ate a lot of fruit got pregnant quicker.[14] This is a very simplified extrapolation of the study, but I think it gives us a nice snapshot of how diet can affect fertility.

Getting pregnant requires a lot of nutrients, vitamins and minerals to keep the very complex chemical pathways firing on all cylinders. Male diet also plays a role because sperm production, count and quality can equally be affected by poor nutrition. The most effective diet for fertility in both men and women is probably the Mediterranean diet.[15] This supplies all the good fibre, vitamins, fats and proteins that are essential for healthy sperm, eggs and a pregnancy overall. Lack of ovulation is the leading cause for female fertility problems and the Mediterranean diet has been shown to help with this, particularly in women with PCOS.[16]

Supplements for fertility

There is an overwhelming number of 'fertility supplements' available, particularly antioxidants. These are compounds that prevent cell damage. It's big business, but there isn't any strong evidence that they actually increase your chances of pregnancy (or decrease your chances of miscarriage).[17] This is why I prefer to tell my patients to focus on getting these nutrients from a healthy diet instead (see Chapter 14). There are, however, some supplements which are worth considering.

Folic acid

Folic acid (vitamin B9) is the only non-negotiable supplement recommended for all women who are trying to conceive. A lot of women tell me they planned their pregnancies, but only started taking folic acid when they had a positive pregnancy test, by which time it might already be getting a bit late. Folic acid helps the body with the rapid cell production that is required in pregnancy and, in particular, helps the healthy development of the brain and nervous system, most of which occurs in the first few weeks when many women don't know they're even pregnant. Deficiency can cause serious neural-tube defects called spina bifida.

Folic acid is a synthetic compound that needs to be broken down for the body to use. Many women are unable to break it down though, so some pregnancy supplements now contain methylfolate, which doesn't require breaking down, making it more available for the body to use. It's been shown to be as effective as standard folic acid.[18] Whichever you choose to take, you should be using it at least three months before trying to conceive to get your stocks up. If you find yourself with a surprise pregnancy, even if you're not sure you want to go ahead, start taking it immediately.

Vitamin D

Vitamin D – 'the sunshine vitamin' – is so important for fertility, as well as bone and heart health. I see so many women who are deficient, but thankfully, it's easy to fix. The NHS currently recommends that everyone should take a supplement from October–March due to lack of sunlight during these months, and this is particularly true for anyone trying to conceive. It's also recommended to use it during pregnancy and breastfeeding, regardless of the time of year. Vitamin D deficiency may hamper the chances of a successful pregnancy, but if your levels are within the normal range, adding even more doesn't provide any extra benefit.[19]

Omega-3

Omega-3 fatty acids are another potentially beneficial supplement when planning a pregnancy. They are thought to play a role in egg quality, ovulation and implantation, and women with lower intakes may take longer to get pregnant. Fish is one of the main dietary sources of omega-3 fatty acids, but I've been seeing more and more women who don't eat fish and are therefore at risk of deficiency. If this is you, then supplementation is recommended.[19] Continuing an omega-3 supplement throughout pregnancy may also reduce the risk of eczema and allergy in your baby.[20] But remember, the biggest benefit is likely to come from omega-3-containing foods, due to the other beneficial nutrients they contain, such as

NEWSFLASH: RED WINE HELPS YOU GET PREGNANT?

A newspaper headline caused a small stir a while ago, stating: 'Red Wine Increases Fertility'. It headed a sensationalised story based on a small study showing that women who drank red wine had higher egg stocks than those drinking spirits or beer. This was attributed to high levels of a nutrient called resveratrol that is found in red grape skins. As an aside, it's also found in blueberries, cranberries, pistachios and chocolate (yay!), which would all be safer sources.

The NHS recommends that pregnant women avoid alcohol completely, and since you won't know you're pregnant for at least a couple of weeks, it's not a bad idea to cut it out while you're trying. A couple of alcoholic drinks per week won't reduce your fertility, but some studies suggest it increases your risk of miscarriage.[21]

There are so many mixed messages when it comes to drinking during pregnancy. It's not helped by the fact that everyone knows someone who went on a bender the night before they found out they were pregnant or drank all the way through their pregnancy. However, there is no known 'safe amount' of alcohol at any stage of pregnancy, from fertilisation right until delivery. Not drinking alcohol for a few months isn't going to harm you, but drinking it might harm your baby. For most people, it's not worth that chance, so I stand by the NHS guidelines and strongly advise against it.

iron, zinc, magnesium and iodine, which are also necessary for a healthy pregnancy.

Caffeine-fuelled eggs?

Caffeine is another thing that we often guzzle with reckless abandon, but I've seen even the most hardened caffeine drinker go cold turkey at the sight of a positive pregnancy test. Although you don't need to be that drastic. The European Food Standards Agency recommends pregnant women drink no more than 200mg caffeine per day – about two cups of coffee or three to four cups of breakfast tea. The same is recommended for people who are trying to get pregnant. Having more has not been shown to decrease fertility, but it is associated with a higher chance of miscarriage.[22] To be honest, I think anyone drinking more than that should probably think about cutting down, regardless of whether they're trying to get pregnant or not. And don't forget that green tea and fizzy drinks are all hidden sources of caffeine. Caffeine is an addictive stimulant that can really affect sleep, and the impact of this on women's health will be discussed later (see Chapter 16).

Exercise and pregnancy

So many women tell me they're not exercising much because they're trying to get pregnant – something that fills me with horror.

Pregnancy puts a massive physical strain on the body. Your heart has to pump more blood than usual to supply the baby as well as yourself, you have to carry an ever-increasing weight and I would describe labour as possibly the toughest workout of your life. With that in mind, ensuring your body is at its fittest and strongest should be a priority when planning a pregnancy. Unless you're overtraining and not resting to the point where your menstrual cycle goes AWOL, you can still do whatever type of exercise you want. It's important to keep active during pregnancy to reduce your risk of pregnancy-induced diabetes and high blood pressure, and it may also reduce the chance of needing a Caesarean section.[23] But during a pregnancy isn't the time to be *starting* new activities, which is another reason why keeping active should be high up on your to-do list of things to do when planning one.

Peeing on a stick – when to do it

You can take a pregnancy test:

- on the first day you miss your period, or
- two weeks after unprotected sex if you don't have regular periods and are concerned about the possibility of a pregnancy, or
- seven days after your period was expected if you have used emergency contraception.

Testing too early gives you a higher chance of getting a false negative (i.e. the test is negative, but you are pregnant) because the test picks up a hormone called human chorionic gonadotropin (hCG), which is detectable in urine about six days after fertilisation.

You do not routinely need to have a blood test. If the urine test says you are pregnant, then you are pregnant. However, it doesn't tell you anything about whether the pregnancy is in the right place or whether it's going to be a healthy ongoing pregnancy. Additionally, a blood test cannot accurately tell you how many weeks pregnant you are, so you will need a scan for that. Please don't waste your money on the expensive tests that supposedly give you this information. They only tell you if you're one to two, two to three or three+ weeks pregnant (which you'll probably already know), and that information will be superseded by the ultrasound, which is much more accurate. I tell all my patients to go and buy a supermarket 'value' pregnancy test, or even one from the pound shop. They're perfectly adequate.

Dating your pregnancy

In hospital, we date a pregnancy from the date of your last period, which can cause massive confusion as it makes you about two weeks more pregnant than you actually are. I've had a lot of awkward moments with patients telling me that I'm wrong because their husbands were away at that time. I recently had to talk a man down from the ceiling when I was scanning his wife and told her she was six weeks pregnant. He sat bolt upright, his eyes wide and told me it wasn't possible. I began to explain how we measure the baby on the screen, but he interrupted me and said, 'No, Doctor, you don't understand . . . she only lost her virginity four weeks ago!' Once I'd calmed him down, he sat back in his chair, smiled and, looking very pleased with himself, informed me that he must have 'amazing swimmers', since he got her pregnant the very first time.

|||||||||||||||||||||||||||||||||||||||||||||

THINGS YOU'VE ALWAYS WANTED TO KNOW, BUT WERE TOO AFRAID TO ASK

What's the best sexual position for trying to conceive?

The one you enjoy! There is no scientific evidence to suggest any one position is more likely to result in pregnancy than another. Also, lying with your bottom/legs up in the air after-wards doesn't help and that's because even just 1 millilitre of semen will contain at least 15 million sperm.

Does female orgasm increase the chance of pregnancy?

As I'm sure you are all aware, male orgasm is pretty non-negotiable if you're trying to conceive. But what about female orgasm? A study suggested that a woman's body holds on to semen more effectively if she orgasms;[24] and of course, the tabloids went wild: *'Reaching climax may raise the chance of conceiving by 15 per cent.'* In my opinion, this was an unhelp-ful piece of research because not only did newspapers make huge claims based on a study of just six women, I also don't like the message it sends to women who are desperate to con-ceive. Not all women orgasm regularly through vaginal sex, and if you've had sex several times in a month it's hard to work out which resulted in conception. Taking these factors into account, it's difficult to really estimate the role of female orgasm in conception from this tiny study, and therefore I don't think it's useful to add this dimension to a potentially already tense time.

How long should I try to get pregnant before I go to see a doctor?

One year. Eight-four per cent of couples conceive within one year, 92 per cent within two years. A lot of couples get quite anxious when it's taking a few months to get pregnant because everyone knows that person who got pregnant the first time they tried, but they are the exception rather than the rule. However, if you're having irregular periods or no periods at all, it is worth seeing your GP sooner to look for easily correctible factors.

I've got a very healthy diet, so do I really need to take a folic acid/folate supplement?

Here is an example of how to get the recommended 400mcg of folic acid per day from your diet:

- Breakfast: avocado (54mcg) on toast with a poached egg (24mcg)
- Lunch: salad containing a handful of spinach (58mcg)
- Dinner: something with a cup of lentils (175mcg) thrown in
- Snack: a handful of peanuts (88mcg)

That sounds pretty easy to do, right? But in the first few weeks of pregnancy? Most people who've ever been pregnant will be laughing in my face right now. The nausea, sickness and downright bizarre food cravings mean that your normal eating habits can go out of the window and I know many women who survived the first few weeks of pregnancy on dry toast, crackers and yoghurts. So even if your diet is on point now, you should really still take a supplement to be on the safe side.

|||||||||||||||||||||||||||||||||||||||||

THE GYNAE GEEK'S KNOWLEDGE BOMBS

There is so much anxiety surrounding fertility. When you start thinking about how many things need to happen for a successful pregnancy it sounds overwhelming. But it doesn't have to be that complicated. Although you don't need to do any specific tests, you should be considering whether your health is in the right place. The goal is to be at your fittest and healthiest at the point of embarking on a pregnancy. Although we are designed to have babies, it does put physical strain on our bodies, so you must optimise the oven before you put the bun inside.

Here's what you need to remember:

○ Not everyone gets pregnant straight away. Eighty-four per cent of couples will conceive within one year of having regular, unprotected sex (twice or three times per week). So for some people it might happen in the first month or two, but it's not unusual to take several months more.

○ There isn't a test to tell you how fertile you are or how much longer you can leave it to get pregnant. There are tests that can give you an idea of your egg stocks, but they're not that accurate. If you do choose to have them done, remember the Pill can affect the results. You should wait three months from stopping the Pill before doing them.

- Folic acid, vitamin D and Omega-3 fatty acids are the only supplements with any rigorous evidence to back up their benefits. There are numerous other 'fertility supplements' on the market, but no strong evidence for any of them, so it's far better to save your money. Instead, focus on a healthy diet full of fruits, veg, healthy fats and lean protein.
- You can still drink caffeine in moderation. Alcohol is a no-no though; there's no known 'safe limit'.

CHAPTER 12

Fertility and egg freezing

*'Could you pass me the salt, please? And also,
I've been meaning to ask you whether you've
frozen your eggs?'*

I've lost count of the number of times I've been asked about egg freezing and, more specifically, whether I have done it. It's often at dinner parties and the table usually goes silent, everyone fascinated to hear what I have to say. While it's a myth that women are becoming less fertile these days, we are having fewer babies because we are starting families later.

The average age for having a first child in the UK is currently around twenty-nine. And around your mid- to late twenties the drunken fancy-dress photos on your social-media feed are slowly but surely replaced with engagement shots and baby photos, and the wedding invitations start to trickle in. And that's when single women far and wide start to wonder about whether they should freeze their eggs. There are also a few medical conditions that can cause problems with fertility, so these may also begin to creep into your thoughts.

This chapter is not aimed at scaring you, rather arming you with the proper facts that can be difficult to come by.

How late is too late?

We are delaying fertility longer than ever at present due to work, finances, difficulty finding the man of our dreams. And that's fine, as long as we all understand that female fertility declines naturally with age from about thirty-two years (see chart below). This is due not only to a decrease in the quantity of eggs, but also in their quality. That's not to say that everyone over the age of thirty-two will struggle to get pregnant – or vice versa; being on the Pill for a decade, for example, doesn't mean you're saving eggs – of course, it's a nice idea, but unfortunately using contraception that stops ovulation (such as the Pill) doesn't prevent the number of eggs from declining at the same rate. Male fertility also declines with age, but at a much less dramatic rate.

This all sounds terribly depressing. Ultimately, you can't fight Mother Nature. But there are some simple ways that you can try and get her on your side, which I covered in the last chapter.

There are also a few gynaecological conditions that might cause problems when it comes to getting pregnant. This is one of the reasons why I think it's so important for women to

MONTHLY FERTILITY RATE BY AGE

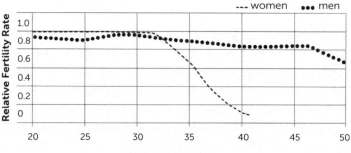

be aware of their gynaecological health and pay attention to any symptoms they may have, so that they can try and get them sorted well in advance of wanting to have a baby.

PCOS and fertility

In my experience, fertility is the single biggest concern among women with PCOS. Yet I often hear women say, 'My doctor told me I had PCOS and would never conceive naturally, so I stopped using contraception and the next month I got pregnant.' That's OK if you want to get pregnant, but it could be a nightmare if not. So please don't stop using contraception if you are diagnosed with PCOS and don't want to start stocking up on this season's must-have maternity wear.

The reason why PCOS can cause problems with fertility is that you don't ovulate regularly. No ovulation, no egg, no chance of pregnancy. In Chapter 4, I gave some suggestions of how to manage your symptoms which may increase your chance of ovulation. There are also medications that can be used to stimulate ovulation for pregnancy. There is a higher chance of having twins using these medications because they turbo-charge your ovaries, so you're likely to release more eggs than you would naturally.

Endometriosis and fertility

Many women are told that the best way to sort out their endometriosis is to get pregnant. The thinking behind this advice is that if you're pregnant, you won't have periods, so you won't get the monthly build-up and bleeding of endometriotic deposits (see page 63), so you shouldn't get as much pain. (This is also the same principle as using the Pill or hormonal coil to manage endo.) It is incredibly unhelpful advice, however, because pregnancy is not a long-term cure for endometriosis; you're likely to have the same symptoms back after you give birth, and – let's be honest – most women don't want to be pregnant most of the time.

But if you have endo, can it impact on your fertility? The answer is yes, for some women, and it is largely dictated by the severity of their endometriosis. Mild endometriosis doesn't normally affect fertility, but moderate and severe endo can decrease your chances of falling pregnant.[25] Medical endometriosis treatment isn't really that effective when it comes to fertility,[26] but surgery often is.[27] That's because the disease can cause scar tissue that distorts your normal anatomy, sometimes preventing the eggs from being released from the ovary, tethering down your fallopian tubes, so they can't pick up eggs and obstructing the way through your tube to your uterus. All these roadblocks stop the sperm and egg from having their hot date, but surgical removal of the scar tissue can free up the route.

Endometriosis is such a complex condition, and severity of symptoms don't always correlate well with how severe the disease is inside your pelvis. This is why you really need to speak to a gynaecologist to determine how you personally may be affected when it comes to fertility, but you can, of course, start trying to have a baby without doing this. I quite often see women who have come to endometriosis clinic to discuss possible surgical treatment having just found out they're pregnant. We happily send them on their way for another year or so to come back after the baby has been born.

Fibroids and fertility

Fibroids, as discussed in Chapter 5, are small overgrowths of the muscle that makes up the wall of the uterus. As well as causing heavy periods, some of them can also cause difficulties when it comes to pregnancy. It's estimated that about 70 per cent of women will have a fibroid at some point, so they're super common,[28] but it's the size, location and number of them that dictate whether or not they negatively impact on the chance of pregnancy. This is because they can change shape of the uterus, its blood supply and the quality of the lining. Again, it's very individual, so you need a chat with a doctor who knows your case to advise you whether a fibroid is going to cause you trouble.

*   *   *

OK, now let's get to the juicy bit that you're all dying to read about . . .

Social egg freezing: a new ice age is approaching

Egg-freezing technologies, or cryopreservation if you want to get scientific about it, was originally developed for young women wishing to save some eggs prior to undergoing cancer treatment that could attack the ovaries resulting in early menopause. Nowadays, many of us take longer to settle down and become financially stable enough to start a family, so using these technologies as a way of delaying motherhood – referred to as 'social egg freezing' – has garnered much interest.

As I've said, your eggs decrease in number and quality as you age, which makes it more difficult to have a baby either naturally or using IVF (*in vitro* fertilisation). There is also a higher risk of miscarriage and chromosomal abnormalities such as Down's syndrome. By freezing your eggs, you stop the egg ageing clock at the point at which they go into the freezer, so if you freeze your eggs at thirty and use them at forty, your risk of miscarriage and genetic abnormalities is the same as a thirty-year-old's.

Advances in freezing and thawing technologies have improved success rates in the last few years and a recently published study showed that they are good enough to result in the same success rates as using fresh eggs for IVF. [29] There is a slightly higher success rate if you freeze an embryo (a fertilised egg), but that requires having also found the man you want to have children with, which the majority of women freezing eggs have not yet done. Alternatively, you could use an anonymous sperm donor either at the point of freezing, or at the point of wanting to defrost your eggs for use.

This sounds incredible . . .

. . . It is, but don't forget that every amazing medical advance comes with its potential downsides. Firstly, there's no guaranteed success. Not every egg will survive, and not every egg that survives will create a good-quality embryo or result in a successful pregnancy. One of the biggest concerns is that women may become too laid-back about their fertility, having frozen their eggs, and could end up without a baby at the end of it. It's never a given.

Secondly, although your eggs are not ageing in the freezer, your body is. The older a pregnant woman is, the higher her chance of developing health complications during the pregnancy, such as pregnancy-induced diabetes, high blood pressure, which can be dangerous for the baby and the mother.

The final drawback, and often the deciding factor for many, is, of course, cost. Social egg freezing is not something that

FERTILITY PRESERVATION FOR MEDICAL REASONS

A cancer diagnosis is the most common medical reason to freeze your eggs. Certain types of chemotherapy drugs may cause infertility, so prior to starting these kinds of medication your oncology team will discuss your options for fertility preservation. Freezing eggs and embryos takes some time and may delay the start of your cancer treatment. If there is a great deal of urgency, it may be possible to perform a short operation to remove some ovarian tissue containing eggs that can be frozen for later use. This may also be used in young girls who haven't started their periods yet.

Women undergoing gender reassignment treatments may also want to freeze their eggs, as the hormones and operations that they undergo can affect fertility. The technique for fertility preservation is largely the same as for social egg freezing. The only difference is the legal limit for how long you can keep your eggs/embryos/ovarian tissue in the freezer; it's ten years for social egg freezing and fifty-five years for a medical reason.

can be done on the NHS and must be funded by your own hard-earned cash. You'll have to pay for tests beforehand, for the egg harvesting, annual storage fee, tests when it comes to wanting to use your eggs and the fertility treatment you'll need to get pregnant.

So how does it work?

You'll need to undergo some blood tests and scans to ensure that egg freezing is safe and likely to be successful for you. Injections are used over about two weeks to stimulate your ovaries to ripen a serious number of eggs for collection. Think of it as a 'turbo-ovulation cocktail'. It's generally safe, but there is a very rare, but potentially dangerous complication called 'ovarian hyperstimulation syndrome' (OHSS).

You'll then need several more scans and blood tests to help decide when your eggs are ready for collection. This is done straight from the ovaries through the wall of your vagina using a small needle under ultrasound guidance. Don't worry, you'll be sedated to lessen the ouch factor. Depending on how many eggs are collected, you might need to do this several times over a number of months. When the time comes for you to use the eggs, you'll need to do ICSI (intracytoplasmic sperm injection) – a special type of IVF where the sperm is injected directly into the egg. It's important to look after your general health if you're freezing your eggs to delay fertility because the healthier you are, the higher your chances of a successful, healthy pregnancy free of complications later down the line.

* * *

If you do think this might be for you, I'd thoroughly recommend going to a fertility clinic to discuss it further – and remember, the earlier you do it, the better the success at the end. Most clinics run informal information sessions where you can go and get more info without any pressure to proceed. Egg freezing is probably one of the most empowering fertility-related advances to date and goes some way towards providing a degree of gender-fertility equality, given that men don't have the same time-related pressures as women.

THINGS YOU'VE ALWAYS WANTED TO KNOW, BUT WERE TOO AFRAID TO ASK

Does egg freezing reduce my natural fertility?

No. Although the medications stimulate lots of eggs to develop, this is similar to what happens naturally every month; it just makes it more efficient, rather than using up the eggs quicker. It hasn't been shown to hasten the menopause. Do remember that it's still a relatively new procedure in healthy women, having been used more extensively in women at risk of undergoing premature menopause. We don't yet truly know whether there are any long-term risks due to the small number of women who have used this type of treatment.

When is the best time to freeze my eggs?

Not too early and not too late! If you already have very low egg stocks, it might not work or you may get very few eggs to store, which is why it's advised to undergo the treatment in your twenties or early to mid-thirties at the latest. It has been suggested that the highest chance of a successful pregnancy can be achieved when freezing eggs before thirty-four years of age.[30] Equally, that doesn't mean that after thirty-four you've left it too late. Unlike a chicken breast, the time in the freezer doesn't affect the quality of the eggs/embryos. However, you're currently allowed to store eggs or embryos for a maximum of ten years in the UK, so you also

182   Part Four: Fertility and Getting Pregnant

don't want to do it too early. If you didn't use the eggs they could be donated for research, training or also for another woman to use.

Would IVF be an option if I can't get pregnant naturally?

Because eggs reduce in number and quality with age, some women find themselves unable to get pregnant naturally or, to put it harshly, they have 'left it too late'. Realistically, most of us won't ever freeze our eggs, so if we found ourselves in this situation, it might still be possible to get pregnant using IVF or similar assisted-reproductive techniques. However, it would likely require the use of a younger donor egg. Over the age of forty-five, most successful pregnancies using IVF are achieved with a donor egg.

|||||||||||||||||||||||||||||||||||||||||||||

THE GYNAE GEEK'S KNOWLEDGE BOMBS

I have found a lot of women to be intrigued by egg freezing, but many don't understand the implications, including the need to have IVF when they actually want to use the eggs, as well as the potential increased risks associated with having a child at an age when their bodies are not naturally meant to do so.

We're very lucky to have these options, but you need to keep your body in tip-top condition if you are planning on delaying your family. Here are the points you need to remember:

o Male and female fertility decrease with age, but it's much more marked in women.

o Underlying gynaecological problems such as PCOS, endometriosis and fibroids can make it more difficult to get pregnant, but it's very individual, so you should speak to a doctor to get a better idea of how you as an individual might be affected. If you have any of these conditions, you should still use contraception if you don't want to have a baby because many women will not struggle to conceive.

o Egg freezing is like an insurance policy: it costs money, might help you in the future, but there is no guaranteed payout.

PART FIVE

Lifestyle and Women's Health

The impact of lifestyle is hugely underappreciated when it comes to women's health. Many diseases and symptoms can have a lifestyle component, and this includes gynaecological cancers. Endometrial cancer is the most common in the UK of the five gynaecological cancers, and 34 per cent of cases could be prevented through lifestyle modification.[1]

It's great to see a huge wave of women becoming interested in improving their health and wellbeing. But I feel many people I come across don't have the right information about how to do this safely and correctly. While I'm still a firm believer in modern medicine, I do think we need to go back to basics and overhaul our lifestyles, not just to improve our gynaecological health, but our general health overall. There are a lot of small tweaks we can make for a profoundly positive impact on gynaecological health and beyond. Because the uterus and ovaries do not function in isolation to the rest of the body. They work in tandem with the brain, the gut and the adrenal glands. I often hear people saying they don't want to put hormones into their body because of the potential health risks (whether these are proven or otherwise). But there is a real lack of awareness of the havoc we wreak with our natural hormones through the way in which we live our daily lives, and of the potential health risks this may pose. Coming to my clinic with a McDonald's burger in your handbag and telling me you always eat really clean is pretty good evidence of this. And yes, that really did happen.

Beliefs about health can also be heavily influenced by non-evidence-based information, (albeit usually well-meaning) on social media. There has also been a shift towards short-term, aesthetics-driven goals, such as the quest for that oh-so-desired six-pack or looking good in a bikini. I want to encourage a more holistic goal and for women to see health as an investment for the long term, so that they are able to enjoy their lives as they wish for many decades to come.

A sensible review of the evidence behind a healthy lifestyle for women is needed, and this is what I aim to cover in this section. I won't provide a 'lifestyle plan'. Humans are incredibly diverse and, as such, I don't believe in a 'one-size-fits-all' plan. What I want to promote is the concept of getting more in tune with your own body and figuring out what's going to work for you.

CHAPTER 13

Stress

'I probably sleep about five hours at best on weekdays, but still manage to make it to the gym four or five times per week . . . coffee sees me through the day . . . and the odd mid-afternoon sweet treat. Work is busy, but I really like my job. So I wouldn't say that I'm stressed . . . '

Stress is usually regarded as a psychological insult that makes us feel upset or anxious, such as a toxic relationship, a looming deadline or financial worries. But actually, stress can result from many factors, such as a lack of quality sleep, always being in 'go-Go-GO' mode, overexercising, too much caffeine and being on a constant yo-yo diet. Developing an understanding of what actually puts stress on your body is the first step in making this link and figuring out what is going to help.

Cortisol is one of the main stress hormones. It's a chemical messenger that tells various parts of the body that something is going on that might require it to react in a variety of ways. Not all stress is bad, and our bodies are designed to expect short bursts of stress (thousands of years ago, this would have helped us escape from a lion, for example). But we are not meant to be under constant stress, which is essentially what twenty-first-century life can be: an ongoing chase from a pack of hungry lions. Constant stimulation of cortisol release and its band of brothers, such as adrenaline and insulin, will have an impact on the production and release of other hormones and, ultimately, your gynaecological health.

So sit back, relax and let me explain why I want you to sit back and relax more often.

The 'brain–vagina axis'?

Many of you will have heard of the term 'HPA axis' (hypothalamic–pituitary–adrenal axis), which is how the brain communicates with the adrenal glands to stimulate production of cortisol (the stress hormone), adrenaline and noradrenaline (the fight-or-flight hormones – remember those lions?) among others. These hormones can then interact with your female hormones. I often simplify this to my patients by calling it the 'brain–vagina axis'. They usually smile and probably think I'm crazy. Then they lean in to hear more.

In an ideal situation, you need a safe, happy environment, with the food, time and resources to grow and raise a child. I've said it before, but I'll say it again: stress acts to shut off your menstrual cycle to prevent you from becoming pregnant. This is an evolutionary mechanism to stop that woman who is being chased by lions, who doesn't have enough food for herself never mind a child, from becoming pregnant. So once your body senses stress, it stops sending the signals to the ovaries that are required for a healthy menstrual cycle. As a result, you will not ovulate or build up your uterine lining in the same way,[2] so that you are less likely to become pregnant. If this stress signal is maintained, it can result in your periods stopping altogether.

Stressful periods

It is well documented that stress has an impact on the menstrual cycle as a result of these changed brain signals, the most extreme examples being seen in studies looking at women affected by war and famine. Although most of us are lucky enough to live in conflict-free zones, our beeping phones, work deadlines, social pressure to be the ideal girlfriend/mother/domestic goddess/social butterfly combined, all while looking like a supermodel, drive the stress response that can start to cause menstrual mayhem. Even social-media use has been associated with higher stress levels.[3]

Many of us have experienced a change in the timing of our period at times of stress, such as an exam or a bereavement. Stress can result in ovulation being delayed. This means that your period is pushed back, arriving late or maybe not at all. Some people also find stress makes their period come earlier.[4] This can be due to a shortening of the luteal phase (the time after ovulation and before your period). It should last about fourteen days, but in women with a 'luteal-phase defect' it can be much shorter due to low progesterone. And one of the reasons that this can happen is because cortisol is made from progesterone. From a survival point of view your body would rather make cortisol because it plays a more crucial role than progesterone. Therefore, if you're churning out cortisol like there's no tomorrow, you'll end up depleting your progesterone stores.

Although not ideal, this isn't generally a problem unless you're trying to get pregnant, in which case a luteal phase shorter than about ten days can be tricky because there may not be enough time or progesterone around for successful implantation of the fertilised egg. It can therefore be a cause of decreased fertility, as well as early miscarriage. If fertility isn't on your radar, it isn't a problem but, 'I'm fed up of bleeding every three weeks and spending all my money on pads and tampons' is something I hear a lot.

Stress also causes the release of prolactin, the breastfeeding hormone.[5] This means your body can get confused about whether you're meant to be breastfeeding or not, and can mess up the timing of ovulation, your cycle in general and whether you have a period at all. It's quite common to see women with slightly high prolactin in clinic and when I ask them if they're stressed they usually say no and tell me the 'poor-sleep, hectic-schedule, no-downtime' tale. (If prolactin is sky-high, milk tends to leak from the breasts, and this is usually down to a small benign tumour in the brain called a prolactinoma, rather than stress. It's quite rare, but it's not a cancer, although it does need to be sorted out to get periods back on track.)

If you're totally stressed out, then the last thing you need is a painful period, but you've guessed it: pain can also be related to stress. I always say that your period is a marker of what's been happening in your body over the last few weeks and months. It's been shown that stress earlier on in the cycle is more likely to make your period more painful, rather than stress closer to the actual event.[6] The same relationship has been shown with PMS: stress early in the cycle can translate to worse symptoms.

One of the biggest concerns with stress altering your menstrual cycle is that it can reduce the amount of oestrogen you make. Having periods which are much lighter than normal can often be a sign that you're not making as much oestrogen. This hormone is very important for muscle and bone strength. Peak bone density is achieved during your late teens and twenties, so if at this time you're not making enough oestrogen you run the risk of thin bones. This can result in fractures from trivial slips and falls, which is more common in women who have gone through the menopause. Young female athletes are known to sustain fractures more easily due to extreme training and not enough food, resulting in low oestrogen production.[7] No one really knows whether this bone strength can be recovered, so if it's happening to you, one of the most important things to do is to ensure you're getting plenty of calcium and vitamin D in your diet. This includes foods such as dairy, oily fish, dark green leafy veggies and soy-based products.

'Just relax and you'll get pregnant'

This is possibly the single most unhelpful comment any woman trying to have a baby could ever receive. However, there is some science behind this well-meaning statement. As I explained above, a stressed-out woman is less likely to ovulate, and if you have no egg, of course, you won't get pregnant. Levels of stress hormone have been shown to be higher in eggs that were not successfully fertilised in IVF, compared to those that were.[8]

It's also important to consider the impact of stress on the father-to-be. Men often aren't as good at admitting they're feeling stressed, and we sometimes underestimate the stress and anxiety that baby-making can put on a man. Male fertility can equally be affected by stress because sperm production is an ongoing, continuous process that also requires hormonal cooperation.[9] The use of psychological treatment has been shown to increase pregnancy rates in couples undergoing IVF,[10] but this is, of course, unusual.

I don't write this to cause any undue extra stress, but I meet a lot of very busy career women who have little understanding of the fact that the way they (and their partners) live their lives could be impacting on their chances of getting pregnant or even just having regular periods. My message is absolutely not 'just relax', but instead, 'do you need to relax more?' And also, to make it quite clear that stress really does have a scientific mechanism.

Discharge can also be stressful, but stress can change your discharge

Bacterial vaginosis and thrush (see Chapter 6) are probably among the most common gynaecological reasons to see a GP. They are often recurrent, with some women getting rid of one bout only to get another the following week. While there are several lifestyle factors that can be associated with these conditions – such as smoking, for example – they can actually be brought on by stress. This may surprise many of you, while others may be nodding their heads – because a lot of people tell me they tend to get BV when they're really stressed or run down. It's is thought to be due to stress-induced changes in the immune system.[11,12]

A thirty-year-old, high-flying London banker I met in clinic a few years ago told me she suffered from terrible recurrent bacterial vaginosis, but that she had noticed it always went away when she went to visit her family in Korea. Upon further questioning, she said she would go there, turn off her phone and emails, sleep better, do daily yoga, stop smoking because her mother didn't approve and drink a fermented soup that her grandma cooked. This may be only one case, but it's a beautiful demonstration of how removing the stress of being a banker in London can affect something so seemingly unrelated as vaginal discharge. (And by the way, I did ask for the soup recipe, but apparently, it's a secret, ancient one!)

One of my favourite ways to unwind is by having a good bath with magnesium salts. Magnesium is best absorbed by the skin, rather than the gut, which for me is a great excuse for a bath – something I previously considered a bit of a luxury, but now see as an essential part of a weekend (always without glasses or contact lenses to ensure that I'm not tempted to try and multi-task by reading a magazine or research paper). I'm also a huge fan of going for a walk without my phone or any music to listen to. And I love a good yoga class.

These are just my personal ideas, but feel free to borrow them or become a bit creative about how you can give your body some quiet time for a few minutes per day.

|||||||||||||||||||||||||||||||||||||||

THINGS YOU'VE ALWAYS WANTED TO KNOW, BUT WERE TOO AFRAID TO ASK

Should we all be meditating?

A lot of patients roll their eyes when I say the word 'meditation'. But the term 'quiet time' doesn't tend to get the same negative response. There are so many brilliant meditation apps, classes and courses out there these days. But for many people the term 'meditation' is offputting because they think it's something that has to happen cross-legged on a yoga mat with a Diptyque Baies candle flickering in the background.

I used to have a habit of listening to music, podcasts or audiobooks when walking, driving or using public transport, as a way of blocking out any stressful or intrusive thoughts when I was feeling particularly anxious. But because we live in such a busy, noisy world, I now ban myself from doing this, even when I'm on my way home from an on-call shift, having been running around for thirteen hours, surrounded

by the constant noise of people talking (sometimes scream-
ing), machines alarming, my bleep going every five minutes
and continuous adrenaline pumping. And it's ironic because
London transport is anything but quiet, but without that extra
level of stimulation, I feel I'm able to use the journey time to
decompress a bit, so that by the time I get home I'm ready
to completely wind down and get a better night's sleep as a
result. I highly recommend that you give it a go, even for just
five minutes, so that you can be quiet with your thoughts.

So while we may not all need to practise formal meditation,
I think there is a lot to be said for ensuring you take some
time to be quiet with your thoughts.

Are my female hormones making me stressed?

They may well be. And that is probably one of the reasons
why women are more likely to have psychiatric disorders
compared to men. While psychological stress and anxiety can
mess with your female hormones, your female hormones can
also cause stress and anxiety. Oestrogen plays a role in the
production and activity of serotonin ('the happy hormone')
and other mood-altering hormones. Too much or too little
oestrogen will alter the balance and can increase depressive
symptoms as well as anxiety.[13] Progesterone can also play a
role in mental health because it's known as the 'calming' hormone, so lower levels can be associated with higher levels
of anxiety, particularly when there is a sudden drop in the
days leading up to your periods.[14] It's a pretty complex situation, but it's one of the reasons why you can notice mood
and anxiety changes throughout your cycle and around the
menopause. For some women, this might just mean they're a
bit snappy in the lead-up to their period, but others may genuinely feel suicidal. This is called PMDD (see Chapter 5) and
as one sufferer once told me, 'This is probably the strangest

thing you've ever heard, but seeing that blood as my period starts is the one thing that calms me down every month.'

Is social media making me stressed?

That's what the studies show. Social media has been rapidly thrust upon us and has dramatically changed the way that we communicate, form new friendships, interact, compare ourselves to others and monitor our self-esteem. High social-media use is not only associated with higher levels of anxiety and depression, but also with body image dissatisfaction.[15] A lot of renowned mental-health experts are quite outspoken about social media being one of the biggest drivers of a rise in mental-health problems, but it's not just people with a diagnosed mental-health problem who are affected: in a study of healthy Facebook users, giving up its use for a week was shown to reduce cortisol levels.[3] While it may not be necessary to do anything that extreme, a weekend away without social media or just turning off the apps for a day or two at a time can really help.

|||||||||||||||||||||||||||||||||||||||||||

THE GYNAE GEEK'S KNOWLEDGE BOMBS

Stress can impact on gynaecological health through several mechanisms, including altering your immune system and the communication between the brain and ovaries, which can manifest as a change in your periods.

Some degree of life-related stress is unavoidable. For many people the source of their stress, such as their job, cannot be removed. Therefore, the most important thing is looking at other areas where stress can be reduced, or where you can ease your foot off the gas to give your body that much-needed release and relaxation. These are the takeaway points from this chapter:

o Stress can alter your menstrual cycle, either by changing the timing of your period, how heavy it is, how painful and how much PMS you might experience. Some people, however, won't experience any change at all.

o Don't feel afraid to have some downtime if you think your hectic lifestyle might be affecting your chances of getting pregnant. There are well-documented links between stress and fertility problems.

o Stress can make you more likely to suffer from thrush and bacterial vaginosis, particularly recurrent episodes.

o Meditation doesn't mean sitting cross-legged and chanting. It's great if you can do it like this, but you could start by simply trying to create some 'quiet time' by getting rid of the constant stimulation of the busy world. This could mean going out for a quick walk without your phone or switching off the radio in your car at the end of a busy day. There are also loads of great apps and online resources when you feel ready to try a more formal form of meditation.

CHAPTER 14

Food

*'I eat takeaways about three or four times a week.
I probably eat fruit a few times a week. But what's
that got to do with my lady issues?'*

Very few people realise the connection between food and women's health. We live in a world where diet culture is pushed into our faces at every opportunity. There is an ever-growing statistic relating to the number of pre-teenage girls who have been on diets, yet the percentage of obese children and adults is also increasing. Then you can flip open your newspaper or scroll through your social-media feed to read about the 'new superfood' and 'The top ten foods for X, Y and Z'. Not to mention the extreme diets for PCOS that I just don't want my impressionable young patients to read, for fear of them developing food fads, or even worse, eating disorders. Where did we lose the plot when it comes to something as seemingly simple as food?

I am no dietician or nutritionist, but prior to becoming a doctor, I did a science degree and subsequently worked in a lab at the University of Leicester, where we conducted research into the anti-inflammatory and anti-cancer mechanisms of brightly coloured plant nutrients called phytonutrients (essentially investigating the science behind #eattherainbow, way before anyone had ever thought of drinking a turmeric latte). And that is where my interest in the link between food and disease was born.

In this chapter, I want to combine my scientific brain, love of food and experience with patients in clinic to explain why food is so important for gynaecological health, but also to show you that it doesn't have to be that complicated. A great tip for starters is to keep a food diary to determine whether there is a link between your diet and any symptoms you experience, and then consider tailoring your diet accordingly to see if it makes you feel better. This should be done in conjunction with professional nutritional advice.

The elephant in the room: weight loss

Most women I meet tell me that they would like to lose weight. And many patients come to me with an expectation that I'm going to tell them to do that. But what's more important than weight is body composition, and this tends to be my focus. As I mentioned in Chapter 5 (see page 59), fat tissue is a source of oestrogen production. Excess oestrogen is responsible for heavy periods, PMS mood swings and also plays a role in the development of many cancers, including endometrial and breast cancer. Excess fat tissue can also increase insulin resistance, which as I explained in Chapter 4 (see page 46) will have a downstream impact on female hormone production as well as increasing the chances of becoming diabetic in the future.

Lean muscle, on the other hand, is very insulin sensitive, and will increase your metabolism, which means it can actually help you to burn that fat tissue that you're trying so desperately to lose. It also gives you more strength to do all the things you want to and enables you to undertake all the strength-based activities that are required to build healthy bones and joints. Therefore, a shift towards a body composed of more lean muscle can provide a healthier environment for happy hormones. Muscle weighs more than fat, however, so some people actually find their weight increases as their body composition shifts. Personally, I am at my heaviest on the scales when I'm at my strongest and leanest. This is one of the reasons I often ignore absolute weight. Plus, it's worth noting that your weight can fluctuate wildly throughout your menstrual cycle, largely due to hormonally driven shifts in water retention, so weighing yourself on a frequent basis will be soul-destroying.

The cravings rollercoaster

Your appetite also shifts with the monthly hormonal roller-coaster; in particular, it has been shown to be often lowest in the days leading up to ovulation and highest prior to that 'time of the month', with more cravings for both sweet and salty foods.[16] Binge-eating, emotional eating and preoccupation with body weight are also highest before your period.[17] With this in mind, going on a strict, restrictive diet is likely to add to the psychological strain of probably feeling hungry (*and* hangry) most of the time. And then you fall off the wagon, you binge, feel guilty, restrict yourself again and the cycle repeats itself.

With all this in mind, plus websites, social media and health professionals giving conflicting advice, what the heck is a girl to eat?

Whole foods: don't over process the basics

'Processed food kills'. I'm sure we've all read that head-line more than once. While I think it is a bit sensationalist, processed foods do often contain hidden ingredients that ramp up the calories and they may have fewer nutrients – so you might eat something that looks healthy, but it isn't as good for you as if you'd made it yourself from scratch. Addressing this could be as simple as switching from a high-sugar breakfast cereal to porridge oats in the morning, or as advanced as making a big veggie-loaded pasta bake with a homemade tomato sauce. Sure, that requires some preparation time, but it's a good way of looking at what's going into your mouth and avoiding hidden sugars, salt and fats. Cooking can also be quite therapeutic, and a lot of patients tell me they really enjoy it because their family don't want to get involved, so they get some quiet time. I find this to be another opportunity for some of my active meditation. But it can also be a way of bringing the family together, and a chance to get children interested in food.

Eat your greens. And all the other colours too

Fruit and veg are an essential part of a healthy lifestyle. We've probably all heard about eating 'five-a-day', and recently it was suggested we should up this to ten-a-day to further decrease our risk of heart disease, stroke, cancer, as well as premature death.[18] The strongest protective associations were seen with green leafy veg, apples, pears and citrus fruits . . . all the colours of the rainbow. That is, in part, due to the phytonutrients: the plant-based nutrients in their colourful flesh and skins which aid chemical processes in the body and provide antioxidants which prevent cell damage.

All these chemicals are crucial for gynaecological health too. It's also worth remembering that ovulation and the menstrual cycle as a whole are complex processes that require a lot of different chemical signals that are made from proteins, sugars, fats, vitamins and minerals. If you're not filling your plate with a variety of colourful foods, you're unlikely to be getting these key ingredients and the whole process will again grind to a halt.

Fruit and vegetable consumption has been shown to reduce the risk of period pain,[19] fibroids,[20] and endometriosis.[21] Many women seem to be afraid of eating fruits with all the 'sugar-is-bad' talk that is going on. However, citrus fruits have been suggested to have the greatest protection against endometriosis, thought to be due to their high levels of betacrytoxanthin, so that means oranges and tangerines, and butternut squash and the humble carrot have high levels too.

Only a quarter of adults in the UK currently consume the recommended five-a-day.[22] That's why my first piece of dietary advice to my patients is to 'try and make every meal as colourful as possible'. They usually look quite intrigued, but many have subsequently told me it's the most fun food-related suggestion they've ever been given. Try, if you can, to find ways to add colour to your meal – for example, by adding a red pepper to your spaghetti Bolognese, or some sweetcorn to your fajitas. Frozen and tinned fruits and vegetables are not only cheaper, but often more convenient when you've got a hectic lifestyle, and don't want to be stressing about working late because there's a carrot in your fridge at home getting more limp by the second.

Female hormones = fat; fat = female hormones

Eating fats is also key for female-hormone production as they're made of cholesterol, which is one of the reasons why a very low-fat diet, or a diet devoid of healthy, unsaturated fats – for example, olive oil, nuts, flaxseed and oily fish, such as salmon – means your body doesn't have the necessary ingredients to make oestrogen and progesterone in the first place. We've become scared of eating fats due to slightly dated dietary advice about a low-fat diet being good for us. Low-fat alternatives usually have more added sugar and sweeteners to make them taste better since the fat has been removed. They often don't contain the same amount of nutrients. Skimmed milk is a prime example, containing fewer fat-soluble vitamins, such as vitamins A and E. I generally prefer to stick to the full-fat option and maybe consider having slightly less of it instead for this reason. A high intake of *saturated* fats should, however, be avoided because they can be associated with higher rates of endometrial and ovarian cancers.[23,24] Butter, processed meats, cakes, ice cream and even coconut oil contain particularly high amounts. But this doesn't mean you should avoid them altogether, especially because they're found in all the fun foods. Instead, enjoy in moderation.

Dairy – don't feel you have to ditch it

I've had so many arguments about dairy and I'm sure they'll continue. At a recent panel event, a very passionate vegan attacked me and my co-speaker, saying we were 'evil for promoting dairy because it ruins our health as well as the environment'. I don't have anything against vegans, but I do have a problem with scaremongering. Many of us are scared to eat dairy and plant-based milks are all the rage these days. And when I ask people why they've ditched dairy they usually frown and say, 'I think it's healthier, isn't it?' Yet there is no solid evidence that there are health benefits to switching to plant-based milks. This means that many women are giving up a precious source of calcium, vitamin D and also iodine (crucial for making thyroid hormones) with no firm reason. While there may be ethical and environmental issues surrounding dairy, you cannot argue with the science: dairy is consistently associated with better health outcomes.[25]

I also come across many people who say, 'But I've heard that dairy causes PCOS because of all the hormones in it.' This is another myth. Dairy does not increase the risk of PCOS, but low-fat dairy may be problematic, and has been shown to increase testosterone levels and prevent ovulation.[26] Acne, which is also hormonally driven and a particular problem in women with PCOS, seems to be more commonly linked with low-fat, rather than with dairy as a whole.[27] So the evidence suggests you shouldn't feel guilty enjoying dairy, but low-fat dairy might be problematic for some women.

'No carbs before Marbs'

'Low-carb' seems to be synonymous with 'healthy diet' and 'weight loss'. However, it's actually neither.

When I ask my patients about their average daily diet many of them throw the question back at me and ask me what *I* eat. Most are surprised when I say my meals are often based around a carbohydrate, such as oats, rice or potatoes (yes, even the white ones!), because carbs have been demonised as an unhealthy food that makes you fat. And a doctor who looks reasonably healthy surely can't be eating lots of carbs, can she? Oh yes, she can!

Carbohydrates are made up of sugar molecules and are the main source of energy for your brain and your muscles in particular. Let's take a ketogenic diet as an extreme example of a low-carb diet, where you eat around 20g carbohydrates per day. A lot of women use this concept before a holiday or wedding. It involves putting your body into starvation mode, so that it is forced to use fat as its main energy source. However, this can actually slow down your metabolism via your thyroid because of the starvation alert it's receiving. Your body therefore tries to conserve energy, you feel sluggish, it messes up production of female hormones, your mood and your periods go haywire – you've heard this somewhere before in this book, haven't you? That's right: a hungry body is not one that makes healthy hormones. You need to focus on getting good-quality, complex carbohydrates into your diet – such as wholegrains (e.g. rice or oats), starches (including the holy potato) and legumes (lentils, beans and peas).

Carbs are also an important source of fibre which, when lacking in the diet, causes . . .

. . . constipation: more fibre and more water, please!

You may be wondering why a gynaecologist is talking about poo. (Numerous 'wrong-hole' jokes spring to mind.) But having a good poo is *so* important for your gynaecological health. Constipation is a massive problem with only 4 per cent of women in the UK currently eating enough fibre.[28] Yet many of us don't realise this because of the vast amount of caffeine we consume which stimulates our bowel, helping us go for a number two.

Fibre is important to keep our healthy gut bugs (microbiome) happy, which is – surprisingly – where a lot of oestrogen production and breakdown goes on.[29] (Wholegrains, including rice and oats, fruits, vegetables, potatoes with their skins on and pulses such as lentils and chickpeas are all excellent sources of fibre.) Becoming constipated can also result in oestrogen build-up because the body can't get rid of it in your poo, so it is recycled around the body. This is bad news for oestrogen-driven problems such as fibroids and endometriosis. Constipation can also exacerbate endometriosis-related pain because your bowel can end up pulling on any scar tissue that's in your pelvis and, particularly if you have endo on your bowel itself, the straining can make the pain even worse.

Chronic constipation can also have an impact on your pelvic-floor muscles, putting them under more frequent strain, causing weakening over the long term. Dehydration is also caused by constipation and a lot of us are not good at drinking enough. I'm always telling patients off when they come to clinic and fish out a fluorescent-yellow urine sample from their handbag. 'You're dehydrated,' I tell them. 'But my urine is always that colour,' they protest. 'Then you're always dehydrated,' I reply. It's only the first wee of the day that should be dark as your body naturally concentrates it overnight. If you're hydrating properly, it should be a very light straw colour the rest of the time. Dehydration is also the commonest cause of daytime tiredness, so it's worth glancing in the toilet next time you pee before you blame *everything* on your hormones.

'She's young – let her eat what she wants . . . '

Healthy food intake is just as important prior to puberty as it is afterwards. Girls who start their periods very early have been shown to be at higher risk of various diseases later in life, including type 2 diabetes, liver and heart disease, as well as hormone-driven cancers, most notably of the breast and ovary.[30-32] Research has explored possible lifestyle factors for early onset of periods and found an association with drinking caffeinated, artificially sweetened soft drinks, thought to be due to the negative impact of caffeine and sweeteners on the brain pathways.[33] Further studies have shown that protein sources may also play a role, with girls who consumed the highest levels of animal protein going through puberty over a year earlier than those who ate mostly plant-based protein.[34] While I certainly don't think it's a reason for young girls to become vegetarians, I do think it is one of many good reasons to be reasonably firm with them about vegetable consumption and limiting fizzy drinks.

WHAT *IS* THE BEST DIET?

The Mediterranean diet is the one style of eating that is consistently found to be associated with numerous health benefits[35] and includes all the good food components I've recommended in this chapter. There are no strict rules, but the principle is a plant-based diet with high consumption of vegetables, legumes, fruits, nuts, wholegrain cereals and olive oil as the main source of fat, moderate amounts of dairy, including yoghurt and cheese, with fish and lean meats and relatively little red meat or processed foods. It's very nutrient-dense and, rather conveniently, it's also been shown to be the easiest to stick to. Compared to the low-carb diet, it's actually better at promoting insulin-sensitivity,[36] which is particularly handy if you've got PCOS and want to spare yourself a life of carb-dodging.

|||||||||||||||||||||||||||||||||||||||||
THINGS YOU'VE ALWAYS WANTED TO KNOW, BUT WERE TOO AFRAID TO ASK

Is it true that veganism makes your periods disappear?
An irresponsible vegan blogger recently claimed that menstruation was a sign of a highly toxic diet, using her statement as an explanation for why vegans often lose their periods: 'If there is nothing to clean, there's no reason to menstruate,' she said. This infuriates me.

Veganism is becoming very fashionable, and I have no problem with people wanting to do it responsibly, with the correct dietary advice from a trained nutrition professional. But the fact is, vegans can become so nutrient deficient that their bodies do not have the resources to menstruate. Zinc, iron, iodine, vitamin B12, and vitamin D are some of the most common deficiencies in vegans,[37] and all are essential for ovulation and a healthy menstrual cycle. If you become vegan – or make any drastic change in your diet – and your period does a runner, make sure you do a runner to a qualified dietician or nutritionist for advice.

I've got endometriosis. Should I cut out dairy?
The evidence says no. In fact, dairy may even be protective against endometriosis. Women consuming dairy three times per week were 18 per cent less likely to develop endometriosis compared to those who had it twice.[38] Vitamin D levels were also lower in women with endometriosis,[38] which is something that I see a lot in my patients. It's thought that vitamin D, as well as calcium, may be the protective factors obtained from dairy. If you genuinely feel your symptoms may be related to dairy, you could try and cut it out. If you

feel better, that's great, but most women tell me they don't actually notice a change. If you do decide to cut it out, do check your vitamin D levels with a simple blood test at your GP surgery and supplement where required.

Is it safe for women to eat soy?

Soy-rich foods include edamame beans, tofu, tempeh, miso, and, of course, soy sauce and soya milk. They contain phyto-oestrogens (plant oestrogens) called isoflavones. While they look similar to human oestrogen, they don't seem to have the same activity. In fact, they actually make a compound called sex-hormone binding globulin, so they have the potential to help mop up excess oestrogen. This is probably one of the reasons why soy intake is actually protective when it comes to oestrogen-related cancers, including endometrial, ovarian and breast cancer.[39,40] Soy may also be helpful for women with PCOS, both improving symptoms and biochemical markers on blood tests.[41] The conclusion? Go forth and eat tofu.

Can certain foods help with bacterial vaginosis?

Deficiencies in vitamins A, C, E, D, beta-carotene and folate can increase the chance of recurrent BV.[42] Should you take a supplement? Not if you're willing to up your veggie game. It's also crucial to look after your gut microbiome by feeding it all the fibre it needs to support your good gut bacteria, because these partly dictate what kind of vaginal bacteria you have. I also recommend my patients to eat plenty of probiotic foods such as Greek yoghurt and fermented foods. Although there aren't any studies to support this concept for the vagina yet, it does work for the gut[43] and it certainly won't do any harm.

||||||||||||||||||||||||||||||||||||||||||||

THE GYNAE GEEK'S KNOWLEDGE BOMBS

We need to think of food as a way of nourishing our bodies, so that they are well equipped to carry out all the essential functions, including making healthy hormones and sustaining a happy menstrual cycle.

Yo-yo dieting and constant restriction are just as damaging as out-of-control intake and emotional eating, so we need something in between. Focusing on calories and macronutrients is exhausting and soul-destroying. Our diets need to be fluid and adaptable, following the ebb and flow of our hormones and busy lives. Some days you might not have a chance to meal prep an Insta-worthy Tupperware, and other days you might want to meet a friend and enjoy a hefty slab of chocolate cake. And that's OK. The most important thing is to find a balance between getting all the healthy ingredients in, but also enjoying the food that you're eating and feeling good as a result.

Here are the key takeaway points for finding a sustainable way of eating your way to health:

- Body weight and weight loss should not be the focus when it comes to thinking about food. Getting the right intake of all the essential nutrients for your body to perform at an optimal level is far more important.

- Eat your fruits and veggies! The health benefits are immense. It doesn't mean you need to turn vegetarian or vegan, but I think we could all manage to up our intake to benefit ourselves.
- A healthy, varied diet largely negates the need for supplements. Vitamin D is the main supplement that is both effective and evidence-based when it comes to women's health. Everyone should supplement in the winter months, and anyone who is deficient should take it all year round.
- If you think there is a particular food/food group that is making you feel unwell or contributing to your symptoms, then firstly keep a food diary to determine whether there really is a pattern, and then consider cutting it out to see if it makes you feel better. But remember you may be at risk of missing out on key nutrients from that particular food, so seek professional nutritional advice.

CHAPTER 15

Exercise

*'Dr Anita, please help me. I haven't had a period
for six months and I don't know why. I'm super-
healthy, eat a really clean diet, go to the gym five
times per week and run 12 miles every
weekend. What can I do?'*

At present I would say I get this kind of message via my
Instagram DMs about five times a week. Exercise is becoming
a huge problem, because there isn't nearly enough awareness
of the impact it can have on our health – both positive and
negative.

And while many women acknowledge the need to be more
active, many don't know where to start. Patients tell me they
can't make it to the gym and therefore can't exercise. But
you absolutely don't have to hit the gym or wear the tight-
est, brightest, most expensive Lycra to be fit and active.
An extreme example of this was demonstrated during a
recent elective Caesarean section theatre session. These are
planned operations and so the atmosphere is usually quite
jovial because there's rarely any urgency or stress, and also
the patient is awake. This particular patient was thirty-two
years old, had diabetes, high blood pressure and a BMI of 56
('normal' is 18.5–25, 'overweight' is 25–30 and over 30 is classified as 'obese'). The anaesthetist was chatting to me about

what I had done in the gym that morning, when the patient piped up from below the drapes: 'Doctor, since you go to the gym a lot, can I ask you a question?'

'Of course!' I said. 'It's one of my favourite topics.' Then, to the scrub nurse: 'Can I have the retractor and another large swab, please?'

'Well,' continued the patient, 'I think I really ought to start doing some exercise, but I have been told it's too dangerous for me to go to the gym because of my weight.'

Needless to say, I nearly fell off my perch (quite literally because I usually stand on a step to operate, being much shorter than most of the surgical staff). Then, once I had composed myself, we had a brilliant chat about how to lead an active lifestyle. It was undeniably one of the most unusual situations in which I've given such advice, but I'm nothing if not an opportunist!

On your marks, get set . . . GO!

Oh wait, false start! I've haven't told you *why* we should exercise.

We all know exercise is 'good for us', but specifically it has been shown to reduce the risk of long-term problems, including diabetes, heart disease, depression and dementia.[44] It can even help with period pain.[45] And sorry to bang the cancer drum again, but regular exercise has also been shown to reduce the risk of endometrial and ovarian cancers. This is not just because of the link between weight and cancers, but also because exercise has been shown to have a positive impact on the chemical pathways involved in cancer prevention.[46] Women also have a higher risk of getting osteoporosis (thin bones), so it's particularly important to be active when we are young because loading our bones and joints is what makes them strong, and that's more difficult to do after the menopause when we might start to see a higher risk of aches, pains and broken bones as a result. Women are also more likely to have hypermobile joints compared to men, so if we can build strong muscles around those joints (such as the knees, shoulders and elbows), we will have a lower risk of joint-related problems.

For many of us, going to the gym is quite simply unthinkable: it's not on our doorstep, it's too expensive, it's full of sweaty men, everyone there is super-fit . . . And I totally understand. It can also be a massive self-confidence issue. I can't count the number of times my friends have asked me to take them to various boutique gym classes in London because they're too scared to go on their own for fear of the fact that they'll struggle, and that everyone else will be parading in their sports bras, looking like supermodels. (As an aside, can I just say that I have trained alongside models and fitness influencers and a lot of them are not as fit as their social-media pages would suggest. And there's a whole lot of #shitloadsoffilter, good lighting and breath-holding going on too.)

When it comes to exercise, I always recommend starting with something simple. Walking is a highly underrated activity – and it's free! While many patients will tell me they don't have time to go to the gym, when I suggest a twenty-minute brisk walk at lunchtime, or even on the way to or from work, most say, 'Oh yes, I can do that . . . but does that count?' The NHS currently recommends 150 minutes of moderate activity per week (enough to slightly take your breath away), so yes – it absolutely counts. I often suggest leaving your phone or headphones behind, so that you can also use it as an opportunity to have some 'you time' and just be quiet with your thoughts. Alternatively, you could try and recruit a friend or colleague to motivate you when you don't want to go. There are two midwives who do this around the hospital car park every morning. They're always deep in conversation, laughing and gossiping away, so it's a pleasure to see.

Public Health England has recently introduced another exercise-related guideline stating that we should all be undertaking 'muscle-strengthening activity' twice a week. This is where it gets interesting, as there are so many to choose from. A frequent question that pops up is 'What's the best kind of strength-building exercise for women?' There isn't a single 'best' form of exercise, and I always tell people to pick what they love and what they're going to stick to. Here are my thoughts on a few types of strength-building exercise that are currently popular.

HIIT it hard?

High-intensity interval training (HIIT) is everywhere at the moment. You pick a few exercises, such as burpees, squat jumps, sprints and push-ups and go hell for leather, alternating for, say, twenty seconds on and then twenty seconds off for several minutes. It's often promoted as the most effective, time-saving workout. And it has been shown to be effective for weight loss, improved cardiovascular fitness and can reduce insulin resistance,[47] which makes it particularly attractive for those with PCOS. It's interesting to note, however, that HIIT training in clinical studies usually involves a seven-to-ten-minute workout, not the forty-five-minute slog that many of us are putting ourselves through several times a week. You can definitely have too much of a good thing.

And when it comes to HIIT, less is more – because excessive exercise will just stress your body out and start to affect your menstrual cycle. A head-to-head study found HIIT and weight-based training to be equally effective for both symptom relief and blood markers in women with PCOS, with neither being better than the other.[48] I'm absolutely not HIIT-bashing, but I wouldn't advise anyone to make it their only form of exercise. Mix it up if you HIIT it up!

#chickswholift

Anyone who follows me on social media will know that I absolutely *love* weightlifting.

It can be overwhelming to go into the weight section of the gym, but you don't have to lift massive barbells if you don't want to. I highly recommend investing in a couple of personal-training sessions, so that you can learn the technique properly and avoid injuries. There are also loads of brilliant classes that include lifting, so this can be a great way to dip your toe in for the first time.

Several doctors have told me that 'weightlifting is not for women'. This is just not true, and I've seen first-hand that many females who lift weights have perfectly healthy menstrual cycles, and certainly don't end up like the Incredible Hulk. Women's bodies are just not designed to become like that, unless really pushed with a specially designed training programme. Anecdotally, my own lifting coach, Adam Willis, and many others in the field, have found that women who don't have periods when coming into the sport find their periods come back within the first few months. While there aren't any scientific studies looking at this yet, I can confidently say I've never heard anyone saying the same about changing their exercise to HIIT training. But again, everything in moderation. And even though weightlifting can make you feel like a total badass, you really don't need to be doing it every day. Mix and match, my friends.

Protect your pelvic floor

One of my bosses at work was horrified when she found out I had started weightlifting; 'Anita, I'm so worried about your pelvic floor!' she exclaimed. And that's around about the time I got serious about pelvic-floor exercises. Pelvic-floor weakness can result in a prolapse, becoming incontinent or problems passing urine or stool in the future.

While there are so many health benefits to be gained from strength training, weightlifting increases the pressure in your abdomen, putting strain on your pelvic floor (as does any kind of impact sport, including running and HIIT training – and, in fact, most other activities we do, including picking up children/shopping bags/suitcases, coughing, even going for a number two). Elite athletes, as well as people who do lots of sport, are known to have higher rates of urinary incontinence due to pelvic-floor weakness,[49,50] but that certainly doesn't mean you should skip the gym. It's just a great reminder that we need to look after all aspects of fitness, including those we can't see, but are going to rely on the most later in life.

Your pelvic floor is part of your core, but you can't train it by doing just any old core exercise, and even if you have the defined abs of a six-pack, you can't guarantee that your pelvic floor is in tip-top condition. I do my Kegels (pelvic-floor exercises) while I'm doing my cool-down stretches in the gym, but it really doesn't matter when or where you do them – it could even be when you're brushing your teeth, stuck in traffic, chopping your veg ... Just don't forget them altogether.

To do pelvic floor exercises, you need to tense, as if you're stopping yourself from doing a wee. (If you're tensing your bottom or thigh muscles at the same time, you're probably cheating!) Hold for three seconds and then release. Repeat ten to fifteen times. Follow this with ten to fifteen short pulses. It might be difficult to start with, but as with all exercises, you'll begin to see an improvement over time. There is a brilliant NHS app called 'Squeezy' (see Resources, page 242) that you can download for more advice and reminders to do them.

An abundance of devices and equipment have come on to the market over the last few years to assist in training your pelvic floor. It's difficult to be sure which are effective and which are a waste of money, so I wouldn't suggest using one without having it recommended by a healthcare professional with experience of using it. Of course, there's nothing better than a real human, and a physiotherapist specialising in women's health is the best person to actually teach you how to do the exercises yourself. And if you've been doing them yourself and it's not working and you're thinking of buying a pelvic-training device, I would still recommend seeing a GP or physio, so that they can examine you to check that your symptoms are indeed related to pelvic-floor weakness.

Yoga isn't just for hippies

I must admit to at first being resistant to trying yoga. I thought it was all just heavy breathing and headstands. Of course, there are many different styles of yoga, some of which can be incredibly strenuous, so it also counts as 'muscle-strengthening exercise', according to the NHS. But as well as helping with strength in general, it also improves core and pelvic-floor strength, as well as balance. It also helps with anxiety, depression, stress and sleep disturbance,[51] due to its ability to tap into the nervous system and the HPA axis (see page 189). There are numerous encouraging studies looking at yoga for period pain and for symptoms of PMS,[52] and therefore I always recommend it to my patients.

Yoga is also helpful for PCOS, but It's tricky to know whether it works purely by its ability to decrease stress and increase pain tolerance, or whether it affects the female hormones directly. However, a very interesting study of girls with PCOS in India found that performing one hour of yoga per day for twelve weeks both improved menstrual regularity as well as hormone markers.[53] For most people, one hour a day isn't achievable, but something is better than nothing. As I see it, it's also 'two-for-the-price-of-one' because you get your strength-training and relaxation done in one, with the potential benefit of your periods potentially becoming less ghastly. Again, there isn't one outstanding style; pick what suits you.

One of the problems I face with recommending yoga is that I think it has become slightly gentrified over the last few years. A lot of my patients think it's something they need to go and do in an expensive whitewashed studio. There are, however, a huge number of brilliant, free YouTube channels with all sorts of types of yoga, so there's something for everyone. My favourites are Yoga with Adriene, and also my friend Shona Vertue (see Resources, page 243).

Hello exercise, bye bye period

I've touched on this topic several times, and I even opened the chapter with it. To be honest, I could probably write a whole book on it, but it would be long, geeky and boring for most of you. So here's my summary . . .

MENSTRUAL CYCLE,
EXERCISE CYCLE?

If you've made it all the way to this point in the book, you'll realise by now that your hormones can impact on various aspects of how your body works. And this applies to exercise too.

During your period, it's been shown that you may perform better at HIIT workouts compared to any other time of the month.[54] This is because of low oestrogen and progesterone levels making you better at mobilising glucose, which is necessary to fuel your muscles for those burpees that you're throwing about. After your period, your oestrogen levels are rising, and you steadily get better and better at building muscle, so this may be the time you want to switch to more strength-based training. If you're lifting and going for a personal best, the time to try is around ovulation when your oestrogen levels peak. After ovulation, you go into the luteal phase and your body gets better at burning fats. This is beneficial for endurance exercise, such as a long run or cycle. At this time, your progesterone is rising, and this can increase your basal body temperature slightly. For some people this makes very sweaty activities kind of uncomfortable, so you might want to stay away from hot yoga or HIIT for fear of turning into an overactive radiator.

You don't need to restrict your activity based on this information, but if you are intrigued, I would recommend tracking your cycle with an app to see if any of this applies. Sometimes it's just nice to know it's not in your head, and that maybe you can't lift as much as last week for a very plausible reason. If you're using hormonal contraception, however, you're unlikely to notice such a drastic change because you won't go through such dramatic hormonal changes as someone who is not.

The reason why excessive exercise will stop your period – known as 'hypothalamic amenorrhoea' – is quite simply because your body thinks you are under attack. It may be that you're putting your body under too much stress, you're exhausted, not relaxing enough, not sleeping well or undereating. Usually it's a combination of all of these. Often, women are told to put on weight to get their periods back. I hate this because I know that if you're someone who is interested in keeping fit, weight gain isn't going to be an acceptable solution.

Many of us want to train like athletes these days, pushing ourselves to the limits and competing with the person next to us, or trying to work out as frequently as that fitness influencer we follow on social media. But right after we finish exercising, we're rushing into the shower, slapping on some make-up while still sweating, inhaling some form of breakfast on the run, working all day with constant stimulation from phones, emails, deadlines, eating lunch at our desks, trying to finish on time, so that we can go out and have a few drinks with our friends, getting home to find there's nothing but hummus and cereal and then spending the rest of the evening scrolling through social media, before suddenly remembering that we need to put our crusty workout gear in the washing machine before going to sleep, often sleeping badly and then waking up exhausted to do it all again the next day. Sound familiar?

Well, it's not familiar to athletes. They train hard, but then they give their bodies time to rest and recover. They take naps. And they eat *a lot*. We all want to be superwoman, but our bodies can only do so much. And something, somewhere has to give. So if you're making your body do all that, it's 'giving' by not giving you your period. If you are very underweight, putting on weight may help. But if you continue to behave in the same way, it's unlikely to do so.

You don't need to stop exercising – and if anyone tells you that, please politely tell them to get lost – but I would advise you to consider the amount and the intensity of what you do. Could you switch a session for something less intense like yoga, swimming or even a walk in the park to catch up with a friend?

And it's not just about the exercise itself, but how you're compensating your body for what you're asking it to do. Are you eating enough? Getting enough downtime to relax? Can you remove any stress-inducing elements in your life? And are you sleeping enough? (See Chapter 16 for the importance of sleep.)

Note: if you feel you're addicted to exercise, this could be the time when you need to go and talk to someone about it. Exercise addiction is a real thing, and if it's happening to you, lack of a period is a pretty strong indicator you need to do something about it.

|||||||||||||||||||||||||||||||||||||||

THINGS YOU'VE ALWAYS WANTED TO KNOW, BUT WERE TOO AFRAID TO ASK

Is it safe to exercise when I'm on my period?

Yes! And it does not cause infertility as a few people have asked me before. Many women feel tired around their period, but it's not usually due to the blood loss so it's not unsafe. The big questions are: do you actually want to exercise? And, if so, what do you want to do? For a lot of people, fear of going to a class or the gym might stem the possibility of leaking everywhere if they've got a heavy flow. Good-quality black leggings are, of course, your friend here. And do remember that exercise doesn't have to be at the gym or structured at all. You could just go for a walk or, if you feel like something more active, put the radio on and jump around your living room. That's one of my favourite activities. Dance like no one is watching and all that! There is also absolutely no shame in taking the opportunity to just have a Netflix marathon in your comfiest PJs; however, some movement can actually be helpful for the pain and also the bloating that a lot of people face.

What's the best exercise for period pain?

A recent study compared various types of physical activity, including yoga/stretching, dance and aerobic activity such as walking, and didn't find one to be better than the other.[45] With this in mind, I say do whatever you fancy. Whatever it is, this study shows there can be merit in trying to do something; it doesn't have to be your toughest, sweatiest workout of the month. Just try and move. Potential mechanisms include increased pelvic blood flow, faster removal of pain-causing prostaglandins from the uterus and increased levels of endorphins (the body's natural painkillers). Ultimately, I don't think it matters whether we find out the precise mechanisms because it seems to help a lot of women and certainly doesn't do any harm.

One thing I will point out, however, is that in most studies, the women performed the exercise all through the month, not just when they were having their period. This is crucial.

As I always say, your period is a marker of what's been going on in your body for the last few weeks. Exercise isn't going to be a quick fix, and it's all about a consistent change for a sustained result.

Is endurance sport dangerous for women?

Endurance sports such as triathlon and marathon running have become increasingly popular and, as with any kind of exercise, they can induce hypothalamic amenorrhoea. As I mentioned in Chapters 4 and 7, the main health risk is that you may not make enough oestrogen, and this puts you at risk of brittle bones in particular. This contributes to the higher risk of stress fractures seen in female athletes compared to men.[7] None of this means that women shouldn't participate in endurance sports – you still have to live your life. But again, it's about making sure you adequately rest and nourish your body. Don't forget to do your pelvic-floor exercises too, because you're likely to be putting them under a lot of strain with long runs. Again, it doesn't mean you shouldn't do it, but prevention is always better than cure.

Is it safe to do a headstand/yoga inversion during my period?

Yes, if you feel able (although some women will be cursing me now for making them even think about moving from the sofa when they're on their period). However, even among hardened yogis, opinions on this topic can be divided. Some say you shouldn't do it because it causes blood stagnation and can make period pain worse because the uterus has to contract harder to push the blood out, since you've forced it in the wrong direction. Some also say it should be avoided when you have low energy and goes against the natural energy flow.

I've also heard the theory that it could cause endometriosis because it could lead to retrograde menstruation, which some say can spread endometriotic deposits into the pelvis. However, other yoga instructors are more than happy to allow their students to do as they feel able. Personally, I don't think there is any decent medical or scientific evidence for either opinion, and particularly not for the endometriosis theory, so I wouldn't specifically advise against it. See how you feel and just go with it.

||||||||||||||||||||||||||||||||||||||||

THE GYNAE GEEK'S KNOWLEDGE BOMBS

Exercise is crucial for health, but you can overdo it. I think we need to look beyond the aesthetic goals and start thinking about the long-term benefits it can have for our health. There's not one single best exercise for women; we are all different. However, we should be doing 150 minutes of moderate activity, plus two sessions of strength-based training per week. This can sound pretty overwhelming, but it shouldn't be a source of further stress in our busy lives, as there are several simple ways that we can sneak it in – such as going for a walk at lunchtime.

These are the main things I want you to remember from this chapter:

- Despite what some people may say, women can weightlift; it's a great way to keep fit and loads your bones and joints to keep them strong for the future. And you needn't end up getting incredibly bulky like the boys. Unless you like that kind of thing.
- Yoga is a multifunctional tool because it builds strength and flexibility, allows you to relax and might even help with period pain and PMS. Try to incorporate it somewhere into your week. There are loads of great YouTube videos you can do in your own home.
- Your menstrual cycle can affect your athletic performance due to the change in hormones throughout the month. You may be interested to track your cycle and see whether this is something you notice in yourself.
- Overexercising can stop your period, but it doesn't mean you need to stop completely when you have it or put on weight. Consider whether you can change your schedule and how you can compensate your body with sleep, rest, relaxation and good food.

CHAPTER 16

Sleep

'I'll sleep when I'm dead . . . '

It's almost time to put this book to bed with a few thoughts about sleep, which is, in my opinion, one of the most undervalued medicines. It's also free. In which case, why do we rate it so little? We've almost come to think of sleep as shameful. No one comes to work and boasts about how much sleep they've had. And heaven forbid you might sneak out of a party early to get your eight hours in. It doesn't help either that countless successful figures and world leaders have openly spoken about 'surviving' on four to five hours per night. Humans are not designed to have such little sleep, and although that may be how we live our lives today, evolution doesn't work that quickly, so we're actually not 'surviving' at all. Quite simply, lack of sleep causes early death and is known to contribute to chronic health problems.

Your menstrual cycle can affect how you sleep, so it's important to consider the need for good sleep hygiene to try and negate some of the impacts of hormones on your sleep. I also use patients' sleep patterns as a way of working out how stressed they might be, as the two can be very much interlinked.

One of the secretaries who types my clinic letters in the hospital once said to me: 'It's really interesting that you always comment on the patients' sleep – why is that?' The other three secretaries in the open office all sat up and started listening and they absolutely lapped up what I told them. 'Wow,' they said. 'It's so important, so why does no one else write about it in their letters?' I'm really not trying to brag here, but I know that many other doctors don't fully appreciate its importance because it's not something we learn about in medical school at all. Thankfully, this information is slowly filtering through and I would like to think that in the future doctors may prescribe sleep because it does have some incredible health benefits.

Sleep is the new sex: are you getting enough?

We tend to think of sleep as a passive existence, where we are not doing anything, which is one of the reasons I think we underappreciate it. In fact, when we sleep, a whole host of genes are turned on, and our bodies set to work repairing things, making hormones and even making memories. The World Health Organization recommends eight hours' sleep per night, but in the UK, most of us are getting between five and seven.[55] Sleep deprivation can make us feel less energetic, lower in mood and our performance at work can suffer, as well as relationships. We've probably all had a cold at some point when we were 'run down' – well, that's because sleep is also essential in maintaining a healthy immune system. But insufficient sleep can have long-term effects too, which include an increased risk of weight gain, mood disorders, memory loss, including dementia, as well as a cancers and heart disease.

Sleep and women's health

I think you know the drill by now: it's time for me to tell you how sleep and female health are interlinked.

A lot of the women I see in clinic sleep terribly. Common reasons for poor sleep include work and financial stress, noise and disturbances from partners or children.[55] For many, awareness that lack of sleep is not great for their health can also add to their stress, which is why I talk about some of the things that you can do to improve sleep (see pages 237–8).

Women with erratic sleep patterns will often report irregular periods. This is because lack of sleep elevates cortisol levels, which – as you probably know by now – feeds back to the brain and alters production of oestrogen and progesterone. Exposure to light when your body isn't expecting it also changes secretion of melatonin, the sleep-inducing hormone, and this again changes your female hormones. Am I sounding like a broken record?

Changes in insulin sensitivity can also be caused by sleep deprivation. Even a single night of four hours' sleep was enough to reduce insulin sensitivity by 25 per cent.[56] This not only means that sleep deprivation could increase your risk of diabetes, but for women with PCOS in whom insulin resistance is a driver of disease, it could be making their symptoms worse. I really want this information to filter down because PCOS can be so tricky to manage, but something as simple as better sleep could have massive benefits.

But your hormones also affect your sleep

Sleep is generally found to be worse in the luteal phase of the menstrual cycle and right before your period.[57] As your body begins to get ready for sleep, your temperature will gradually drop as one of the signs that it's time to go to sleep. This drop continues, becoming its lowest during the night when you're normally asleep. The temperature change isn't usually enough for you to notice if you're following your usual sleep pattern, but if you've ever wondered why you feel cold when you're really tired at night, this is the reason why. Get yourself to bed, pronto! However, in the luteal phase your temperature will usually be ever so slightly higher. Again, not often enough for you to notice, but some people find themselves way too hot at night, even waking up in pools of sweat, which can disrupt their sleep as a result. If your temperature is higher, you may also not feel as sleepy at bedtime compared to earlier in your cycle. One tip here is to make sure that your bedroom is cool enough (aim for about 18°C) and that you don't have too many covers on.

The sudden drop in progesterone right before your period can also affect sleep since progesterone is known to be the calming hormone and promotes melatonin production.[58] So when you've got less of it, your sleep may be worse. During this entire phase, your sleep can generally be more fragmented. It doesn't necessarily mean that you'll wake up in the middle of the night and remember it, but you are more likely to have very vivid or bizarre dreams.

Given all these factors, it's not surprising that PMS and PMDD (see pages 65–6) can be made worse by sleep deprivation.[59]

When your period finally comes, the cramps might keep you awake. A lot of people say their period pains are worse at night. It's been suggested that this is because lying in a horizontal position means your uterus has to squeeze more to try and get the blood out, although this is refuted by those who say it isn't actually worse – it's just that there's nothing to distract us from the pain like there is in the day.

Thankfully, as your period finishes, oestrogen levels start

to rise and sleep generally improves, so make the most of it!

I highly recommend tracking your cycle to see how it affects your sleep. You can then use this information to try and prioritise sleep-promoting activities at the relevant times. Taking the contraceptive Pill can attenuate many of these changes, so you might not notice the same effects. It does slightly elevate your basal body temperature, but has not been shown to alter sleep quality overall.[60]

Tired and wired . . . too much coffee?

Caffeine is one of the most overused drugs and is a real cause of poor sleep. It can be great for waking you up and improving concentration, and coffee consumption can even have health benefits such as a decreased risk of heart disease.[61] However, all these happen at a low dose. Drinking too much coffee can leave you jittery, unable to concentrate, anxious and, most of all, unable to sleep.

Caffeine works by blocking adenosine receptors. Adenosine is a chemical that tells us we are sleepy. So if your coffee is sat in its place, your body doesn't realise you're tired and won't send the right sleep-promoting signals. It doesn't replace the need for sleep though. You also get a release of adrenaline, the fight-or-flight hormone, and cortisol. And, as we saw earlier (see p. 00), these can impact on production of female hormones. A daily caffeine consumption greater than 300mg (approximately three cups of coffee) has been associated with a shorter menstrual cycle, as well as fewer days of bleeding,[62] which supports the theory that caffeine consumption does affect your hormones. It's also been shown that high caffeine consumption can result in an earlier menopause,[63] which increases the chance of osteoporosis and heart disease.

Remember too that decaffeinated coffee is never entirely caffeine-free, so bear that in mind if you're swigging it before bed. Always check fizzy drinks, and note that green tea also contains caffeine (I have a lot of patients who drink it like water), although I recently heard a great tip to reduce the amount of caffeine in your green tea, by making it with hot, not boiling water; so that's worth a try if you're a massive green-tea fan. Some headache tablets and painkillers also contain caffeine. It's usually the ones with 'plus' at the end of their names. I never buy them. They are no more effective, and I don't want to end up having a sleepless night with heart palpitations from a late-night caffeine hit when all I did, bleary-eyed, was reach for a paracetamol when I had period pain.

A final, slightly unrelated fact about caffeine is that it can cause bladder irritability, so if you're always dashing to the loo, either day or night, consider your caffeine intake.

In summary, enjoy in moderation, and always before twelve noon, so that you have time to excrete the majority of the caffeine before bedtime for a restful night.

Alcohol: I don't mean to be a party pooper, but . . .

Twenty per cent of women are said to admit to using alcohol to help them get to sleep,[55] but from what people tell me, I feel this figure should be higher. Either way, using alcohol to promote sleep is a real mistake. While it may help you get to sleep quicker, it will result in poorer-quality sleep, due to a lack of deep sleep, which is when your body undertakes its necessary restorative processes. So you'll spend more time in a lighter phase of sleep, which, although part of the normal sleep cycle, will result in a more restless night, often causing you to wake several times. You might also have some odd dreams or even nightmares. Don't forget that alcohol is also a diuretic, which is why you often wake up with a bladder that's about to burst and a mouth that's drier than the Sahara.

The jury is still out regarding whether alcohol impacts

BLUE LIGHT

Smartphones and tablets are probably the best and worst inventions when it comes to a busy life. It's great that we have everything at our fingertips at the flick of a switch, but it also means we can be constantly at work when we're meant to be at home relaxing. (How easy is it to waste an entire evening scrolling through social media!) And these things will keep us stimulated, fired up and in 'On' mode, which, of course, make it more difficult to sleep. But the artificial blue light that is emitted from the screens that we hold so closely to our faces also confuses the brain and makes us think we are being exposed to sunlight. In turn, we produce less melatonin, and it becomes difficult to fall asleep, even when we are completely exhausted.

I suggest investing in a good old-fashioned alarm clock, so that you can leave temptation (the phone) out of the bedroom, and sleep soundly. In fact, along with many sleep experts, I highly recommend a 'digital detox' before bed. Ideally, it should be about ninety minutes before, but you could even just start with twenty. It will allow your brain to start to switch off and tell your body that it's time to go to bed; that way, you are likely to find that you sleep much better.

your menstrual cycle and, if so, to what extent. This is probably because of the huge number of variables, ranging from the types of alcohol consumed to the different circumstances in which people drink – say, acute stress or celebration. What is interesting, however, is that your cycle can dictate whether you want to drink or not. A desire to drink has been shown to be stronger in the luteal phase, the time after ovulation and before your period, which is the same time that the depressive symptoms associated with alcohol can also be greater.[64] And many women will attest to the fact that PMS drives them to drink: 'My period is due and all I want to do is sit on the sofa and polish off a bottle of wine!' But although it hasn't been confirmed whether it makes your PMS worse, there are far more constructive ways to deal with it, such as physical activity, which will definitely help your sleep – as remember, lack of sleep can make your PMS worse. It's all a vicious cycle!

Drinking is quite heavily ingrained in our society, although an increasing number of people are cutting down on alcohol or even becoming teetotal. I don't normally shout about the fact that I don't drink alcohol very much any more, but a surprising number of people have admitted to me that they'd also rather not drink sometimes, but feel a certain amount of social pressure to do so. If you can say no to having that extra helping of food, you can do the same when it comes to alcohol. It doesn't make you less fun, and it might just help you sleep better.

Sleep hygiene

People often tell me, 'I don't really sleep well in the week because I'm out most nights. But then I try and have a really long lie-in on the weekends.' Unfortunately, it's quite difficult to pay back a sleep debt in this way. That's because even one night of limited sleep can have a profound effect on the chemical signals going around the brain, on our immune systems and our hormones. Therefore, it's important to try and keep things even over the whole week. If you're having an erratic sleep pattern with different bedtimes and morning alarms, your body will easily be confused, and you end up spending your entire time with what is essentially 'social jet lag'. Of course, there will always be times when you can't avoid a late night or a horribly early morning, but try and keep these to a minimum.

If you've noticed that you don't tend to sleep as well when you're coming up to your period, it's even more important to try and have a good bedtime routine. Anxiety levels can also be higher in the premenstrual phase, so this really is the time to prioritise a good wind-down, such as pre-bed meditation, yoga, reading a book or listening to music. Keeping your bedroom cool and as dark as possible, without the little LED lights from TV and other electronic devices will also help.

|||||||||||||||||||||||||||||||||||||||||

THINGS YOU'VE ALWAYS WANTED TO KNOW, BUT WERE TOO AFRAID TO ASK

Why does travel/jet lag mess with my periods?

Have you ever been on a trip and found your period was later or earlier than usual? This is a totally normal phenomenon that occurs as a result of jet lag: the fatigue experienced from travelling across time zones. It is largely because of the impact it has on levels of the sleep hormone, melatonin, which will be altered by exposure to light at a different time. Changes in melatonin production have a knock-on effect on the brain's production of those hormones that signal to the ovaries. A similar phenomenon is seen in people who do night shifts, which is much like jet lag, but without the promise of a sunbed and a tropical cocktail at the end of it!

It can make it difficult to track your fertile window during periods of travel, which is why using fertility-awareness methods of contraception can be tricky in this situation, and I've seen a lot of women who've got pregnant as a result (see pages 102–3 and 161–2 for more on fertility-awareness contraception).

Is social media affecting my sleep?

It may well be. We've all decided to 'have a quick scroll' and found ourselves an hour later looking through the account of someone we don't even know or follow. Social-media use not only encroaches on the time available to sleep, but exposes us to blue light before bed. It's also been shown that using social media increases anxiety, which also negatively impacts on sleep quality.[65] Don't be afraid to unfollow accounts that don't make you feel good about yourself and try and enforce a 'digital detox' as part of your bedtime regime.

Is late-night exercise ruining my sleep?

Exercising late at night can stop you from getting that much-needed quality sleep. A lot of the women I see love going to a super-sweaty gym class in the evening or for a long run not long before bed to blow off some steam and get rid of the stress of the day. That can, however, result in becoming more awake afterwards at a time when the body is trying to wind down. A study of elite athletes showed that performing a six-minute mindfulness exercise before bed improved sleep quality after night-time training,[66] so this could be something to try if your schedule only permits evening exercise, or if it's just your preferred time.

Should I track my sleep?

There's an app for everything these days, and of course there are loads of apps and wearable devices available to track your sleep. This can be handy to give you a generalised picture of how well you're doing and can be useful in providing some positive reinforcement that sleeping more really is making you feel better. However, there is a phenomenon known as 'orthosomnia' which is a preoccupation with improving sleep data using trackers,[67] so don't get too obsessed. Remember, how you feel is much more important than how a screen tells you that you should feel.

||||||||||||||||||||||||||||||||||||||||

THE GYNAE GEEK'S KNOWLEDGE BOMBS

Sleep is free and it makes you live a longer, happier life. But it's not something we were taught about at medical school and, to be honest, it took me a while to realise its importance. It doesn't matter how healthy your diet is, or however else you take care of yourself – sleep cannot be replaced by anything else. Although handily, if you are nailing the other basics – good diet, keeping active and relaxed – you're much more likely to sleep better. I hope I've managed to convince you that a lack of sleep can be detrimental to women's health, and that there is a huge interplay between the two, as well as between the common disruptors.

Here are the key points to remember from this chapter:

- Your menstrual cycle can affect your sleep. Sleep is most commonly disturbed after ovulation and in the lead-up to your period due to changes in core body temperature and progesterone levels.
- Wind-down time is a great way to get ready for a better sleep and might be even more important at the times of the month when you feel your sleep is most disrupted. This could involve switching off electronic devices because of the negative impact of blue light on your sleep hormone production.
- A sleep debt can be difficult to repay. Try and maintain a sleep routine throughout the week, rather than trying to compensate with a lie-in at the weekend.
- Caffeine and alcohol are two major sleep disruptors. You don't have to go cold turkey, but enjoy them sensibly and think quality over quantity when you do so.

Final thoughts

I've snatched every spare moment over the last few months to sit down and write. I've written in the back of the car, on the London Underground and on planes, in conference halls and on the beach, in London and Dubrovnik, in the middle of the night in the labour ward on-call room and from my bed when I've been unable to get up due to a tough shift at work the day before.

You may ask why I put myself through all that. And the answer is that I saw a desperate need for women to get basic information about female health. I've seen women who were unsure about whether their symptoms were normal; women too embarrassed to go and speak to their doctors about their female health; women who did not know what to call their 'bits'; women who broke down in front of me because Dr Google had diagnosed them with all sorts of dreadful diseases (that they absolutely didn't have); women who were being misled by unqualified folk on social media; and I saw the damage that women were doing to their gynaecological health through their hectic lifestyles.

As a final refresher from these pages, here are sixteen key things that every woman needs to know:

- Your vulva is on the outside and your vagina is on the inside.

- Your labia are supposed to be visible from the outside and are normally uneven in shape and size. Don't let anyone tell you they need to be trimmed to 'neaten them up' and make them symmetrical.
- The average menstrual cycle lasts twenty-eight days, although anything from twenty-one to thirty-five days is considered 'normal'. Day 1 is the first day of your period.
- Polycystic ovarian syndrome (PCOS) is a common cause of irregular periods. It doesn't have to be a life sentence and there are a lot of lifestyle changes that can be implemented for a potentially profound effect on your symptoms.
- There are many reasons for heavy and painful periods that are very treatable, so it's not something that you have to 'put up with'. Cancer is the thing that everyone with these symptoms worries about, but it's actually one of the rarest causes.
- Vaginal discharge is the reason you exist. It's there to protect you. You need to learn what's normal before you can work out what's abnormal.
- The withdrawal method is not a reliable form of contraception. Don't use it.
- Using emergency contraception does not cause an abortion, and abortions do not make you infertile.
- Sexually transmitted diseases, on the other hand, *can* affect your fertility. And if you've never been tested, you can't be certain that you've never had one.
- Smear testing is the best way of preventing cervical cancer. And pretty much everyone gets HPV, which is the virus that causes it, although it usually goes away fairly quickly and doesn't cause any problems. It's not a sign of promiscuity.
- You don't need any kind of fertility test before trying to

get pregnant. In most cases they won't tell you anything useful and they are not that reliable.

○ Egg freezing is a way of preserving your fertility until you're ready to have children, but it's not 100 per cent guaranteed.

○ Stress can come in many forms and can affect your menstrual cycle – because Mother Nature never intended for a stressed-out woman to get pregnant in case she is unable to protect her child.

○ You are what you eat. Food choices can have a massive impact on female health.

○ When it comes to exercise you *can* have too much of a good thing. And if overexercising stops your periods, it can have a negative impact on your health for the future, and could increase your risk of thin bones in older age.

○ Sleep is the most underrated medicine.

If any of the information in this book has worried you, or you think you may have a problem that requires further attention, I hope that you will feel empowered, and maybe less embarrassed or anxious to go and speak to your doctor.

Please value your body. Remember, it's the only one you've got, so you need to look after it. No one wants to think about getting old, but it's inevitable, so we all need to implement a healthy lifestyle today as an investment for the future.

Resources

Health apps

Clue app – to track your menstrual cycle
    https://helloclue.com

Moody Month app – to track your menstrual cycle and both mental and physical hormone-related symptoms
    https://moodymonth.com/

Squeezy app – for pelvic floor exercise reminders and advice
    https://www.squeezyapp.com/

Doctors to follow for lifestyle advice

Dr Rupy Aujla (@thedoctorskitchen) – for plant-based recipes and a health and lifestyle podcast
    https://thedoctorskitchen.com/

Dr Rangan Chatterjee (@drchatterjee) – a podcast talking about lifestyle medicine
    https://drchatterjee.com/

Dr Hazel Wallace (@thefoodmedic) – for healthy recipes, workouts and a health and wellbeing podcast
    https://thefoodmedic.co.uk/

Websites

SH:24 is a free online sexual-health service
  https://www.sh24.org.uk/

My favourite YouTube Yoga channels

Shona Vertue
  http://shonavertue.com
  https://www.youtube.com/channel UCw3_asTSehMF-MbF1
    cluGCw

Yoga with Adriene
  https://yogawithadriene.com
  https://www.youtube.com/user/yogawithadriene

Notes

Part One

1. Lloyd J, Crouch NS, Minto CL, Liao LM, Creighton SM. Female genital appearance: "normality" unfolds. *BJOG* 2005; **112**(5): 643–6.
2. Rowen TS, Gaither TW, Awad MA, Osterberg EC, Shindel AW, Breyer BN. Pubic Hair Grooming Prevalence and Motivation Among Women in the United States. *JAMA Dermatol* 2016; **152**(10): 1106–13.
3. Schreiner L, Crivelatti I, de Oliveira JM, Nygaard CC, Dos Santos TG. Systematic review of pelvic floor interventions during pregnancy. *Int J Gynaecol Obstet* 2018.
4. Woodley SJ, Boyle R, Cody JD, Morkved S, Hay-Smith EJC. Pelvic floor muscle training for prevention and treatment of urinary and faecal incontinence in antenatal and postnatal women. *Cochrane Database Syst Rev* 2017; **12**: CD007471.
5. Younis MT, Iram S, Anwar B, Ewies AA. Women with asymptomatic cervical polyps may not need to see a gynaecologist or have them removed: an observational retrospective study of 1126 cases. *Eur J Obstet Gynecol Reprod Biol* 2010; **150**(2): 190–4.
6. Tarney CM, Han J. Postcoital bleeding: a review on etiology, diagnosis, and management. *Obstet Gynecol Int* 2014; **2014**: 192087.
7. Royal College of Obstetricians & Gynaecologists. Ovarian Masses in Premenopausal Women, Management of Suspected (Green-top Guideline No. 62). 2011.
8. Parkin DM, Boyd L, Walker LC. 16. The fraction of cancer attributable to lifestyle and environmental factors in the UK in 2010. *Br J Cancer* 2011; **105 Suppl 2**: S77–81.

Part Two

1. Johnson S, Marriott L, Zinaman M. Can apps and calendar methods predict ovulation with accuracy? *Curr Med Res Opin* 2018: 1–18.
2. Dasharathy SS, Mumford SL, Pollack AZ, et al. Menstrual bleeding patterns among regularly menstruating women. *Am J Epidemiol* 2012; **175**(6): 536–45.
3. Cole LA, Ladner DG, Byrn FW. The normal variabilities of the menstrual cycle. *Fertil Steril* 2009; **91**(2): 522–7.
4. Howard C, Rose CL, Trouton K, et al. FLOW (finding lasting options for women): multicentre randomized controlled trial comparing tampons with menstrual cups. *Can Fam Physician* 2011; **57**(6): e208–15.
5. Meaddough EL, Olive DL, Gallup P, Perlin M, Kliman HJ. Sexual activity, orgasm and tampon use are associated with a decreased risk for endometriosis. *Gynecol Obstet Invest* 2002; **53**(3): 163–9.
6. Mitchell MA, Bisch S, Arntfield S, Hosseini-Moghaddam SM. A confirmed case of toxic shock syndrome associated with the use of a menstrual cup. *Can J Infect Dis Med Microbiol* 2015; **26**(4): 218–20.
7. Archer JC, Mabry-Smith R, Shojaee S, Threet J, Eckert JJ, Litman VE. Dioxin and furan levels found in tampons. *J Womens Health (Larchmt)* 2005; **14**(4): 311–5.
8. DeVito MJ, Schecter A. Exposure assessment to dioxins from the use of tampons and diapers. *Environ Health Perspect* 2002; **110**(1): 23–8.
9. Strotmeyer ES, Steenkiste AR, Foley TP, Jr., Berga SL, Dorman JS. Menstrual cycle differences between women with type 1 diabetes and women without diabetes. *Diabetes Care* 2003; **26**(4): 1016–21.
10. Solomon CG, Hu FB, Dunaif A, et al. Long or highly irregular menstrual cycles as a marker for risk of type 2 diabetes mellitus. *JAMA* 2001; **286**(19): 2421–6.
11. Teede H, Deeks A, Moran L. Polycystic ovary syndrome: a complex condition with psychological, reproductive and metabolic manifestations that impacts on health across the lifespan. *BMC Med* 2010; **8**: 41.
12. Mavropoulos JC, Yancy WS, Hepburn J, Westman EC. The effects of a low-carbohydrate, ketogenic diet on the polycystic ovary syndrome: a pilot study. *Nutr Metab (Lond)* 2005; **2**: 35.
13. Lee I, Cooney LG, Saini S, et al. Increased risk of disordered eating in polycystic ovary syndrome. *Fertil Steril* 2017; **107**(3): 796–802.

14. Eslamian G, Baghestani AR, Eghtesad S, Hekmatdoost A. Dietary carbohydrate composition is associated with polycystic ovary syndrome: a case-control study. *J Hum Nutr Diet* 2017; **30**(1): 90–7.
15. Cooney LG, Lee I, Sammel MD, Dokras A. High prevalence of moderate and severe depressive and anxiety symptoms in polycystic ovary syndrome: a systematic review and meta-analysis. *Hum Reprod* 2017; **32**(5): 1075–91.
16. Naderpoor N, Shorakae S, de Courten B, Misso ML, Moran LJ, Teede HJ. Metformin and lifestyle modification in polycystic ovary syndrome: systematic review and meta-analysis. *Hum Reprod Update* 2016; **22**(3).
17. Pundir J, Psaroudakis D, Savnur P, et al. Inositol treatment of anovulation in women with polycystic ovary syndrome: a meta-analysis of randomised trials. *BJOG* 2018; **125**(3): 299–308.
18. Metcalf MG, Skidmore DS, Lowry GF, Mackenzie JA. Incidence of ovulation in the years after the menarche. *J Endocrinol* 1983; **97**(2): 213–9.
19. Harris HR, Titus LJ, Cramer DW, Terry KL. Long and irregular menstrual cycles, polycystic ovary syndrome, and ovarian cancer risk in a population-based case-control study. *Int J Cancer* 2017; **140**(2): 285–91.
20. Harris HR, Terry KL. Polycystic ovary syndrome and risk of endometrial, ovarian, and breast cancer: a systematic review. *Fertil Res Pract* 2016; **2**: 14.
21. Friberg E, Mantzoros CS, Wolk A. Diabetes and risk of endometrial cancer: a population-based prospective cohort study. *Cancer Epidemiol Biomarkers Prev* 2007; **16**(2): 276–80.
22. Voskuil DW, Monninkhof EM, Elias SG, et al. Physical activity and endometrial cancer risk, a systematic review of current evidence. *Cancer Epidemiol Biomarkers Prev* 2007; **16**(4): 639–48.
23. Polson DW, Adams J, Wadsworth J, Franks S. Polycystic ovaries – a common finding in normal women. *Lancet* 1988; **1**(8590): 870–2.
24. Fraser IS, Warner P, Marantos PA. Estimating menstrual blood loss in women with normal and excessive menstrual fluid volume. *Obstet Gynecol* 2001; **98**(5 Pt 1): 806–14.
25. Duckitt K, Collins S. Menorrhagia. *BMJ Clin Evid* 2008; **2008**.
26. Zahradnik HP, Hanjalic-Beck A, Groth K. Nonsteroidal anti-inflammatory drugs and hormonal contraceptives for pain relief from dysmenorrhea: a review. *Contraception* 2010; **81**(3): 185–96.
27. Marjoribanks J, Ayeleke RO, Farquhar C, Proctor M. Nonsteroidal anti-inflammatory drugs for dysmenorrhoea. *Cochrane Database Syst Rev* 2015; (7): CD001751.

28. Dehnavi ZM, Jafarnejad F, Kamali Z. The Effect of aerobic exercise on primary dysmenorrhea: A clinical trial study. *J Educ Health Promot* 2018; **7**: 3.
29. Kikuchi H, Nakatani Y, Seki Y, et al. Decreased blood serotonin in the premenstrual phase enhances negative mood in healthy women. *J Psychosom Obstet Gynaecol* 2010; **31**(2): 83–9.
30. Lanza di Scalea T, Pearlstein T. Premenstrual Dysphoric Disorder. *Psychiatr Clin North Am* 2017; **40**(2): 201–16.
31. Pennant ME, Mehta R, Moody P, et al. Premenopausal abnormal uterine bleeding and risk of endometrial cancer. *BJOG* 2017; **124**(3): 404–11.
32. Pattanittum P, Kunyanone N, Brown J, et al. Dietary supplements for dysmenorrhoea. *Cochrane Database Syst Rev* 2016; **3**: CD002124.

Part Three

1. McCann MF, Irwin DE, Walton LA, Hulka BS, Morton JL, Axelrad CM. Nicotine and cotinine in the cervical mucus of smokers, passive smokers, and nonsmokers. *Cancer Epidemiol Biomarkers Prev* 1992; **1**(2): 125–9.
2. Windham GC, Mitchell P, Anderson M, Lasley BL. Cigarette smoking and effects on hormone function in premenopausal women. *Environ Health Perspect* 2005; **113**(10): 1285–90.
3. Law MR, Hackshaw AK. A meta-analysis of cigarette smoking, bone mineral density and risk of hip fracture: recognition of a major effect. *BMJ* 1997; **315**(7112): 841–6.
4. Brotman RM, He X, Gajer P, et al. Association between cigarette smoking and the vaginal microbiota: a pilot study. *BMC Infect Dis* 2014; **14**: 471.
5. Darvishi M, Jahdi F, Hamzegardeshi Z, Goodarzi S, Vahedi M. The Comparison of vaginal cream of mixing yogurt, honey and clotrimazole on symptoms of vaginal candidiasis. *Glob J Health Sci* 2015; **7**(6): 108–16.
6. Bisschop MP, Merkus JM, Scheygrond H, van Cutsem J. Co-treatment of the male partner in vaginal candidosis: a double-blind randomized control study. *Br J Obstet Gynaecol* 1986; **93**(1): 79–81.
7. Foxman B, Muraglia R, Dietz JP, Sobel JD, Wagner J. Prevalence of recurrent vulvovaginal candidiasis in 5 European countries and the United States: results from an internet panel survey. *J Low Genit Tract Dis* 2013; **17**(3): 340–5.
8. Xie HY, Feng D, Wei DM, et al. Probiotics for vulvovaginal

candidiasis in non-pregnant women. *Cochrane Database Syst Rev* 2017; **11**: CD010496.

9. Brotman RM, Shardell MD, Gajer P, et al. Association between the vaginal microbiota, menopause status, and signs of vulvovaginal atrophy. *Menopause* 2014; **21**(5): 450–8.
10. Larsson PG. Treatment of bacterial vaginosis. *Int J STD AIDS* 1992; **3**(4): 239–47.
11. Homayouni A, Bastani P, Ziyadi S, et al. Effects of probiotics on the recurrence of bacterial vaginosis: a review. *J Low Genit Tract Dis* 2014; **18**(1): 79–86.
12. Amaya-Guio J, Viveros-Carreno DA, Sierra-Barrios EM, Martinez-Velasquez MY, Grillo-Ardila CF. Antibiotic treatment for the sexual partners of women with bacterial vaginosis. *Cochrane Database Syst Rev* 2016; **10**: CD011701.
13. Ogbolu DO, Oni AA, Daini OA, Oloko AP. In vitro antimicrobial properties of coconut oil on Candida species in Ibadan, Nigeria. *J Med Food* 2007; **10**(2): 384–7.
14. te Velde ER, Eijkemans R, Habbema HD. Variation in couple fecundity and time to pregnancy, an essential concept in human reproduction. *Lancet* 2000; **355**(9219): 1928–9.
15. World Health Organization. WHO Model Lists of Essential Medicines. 2017. http://www.who.int/medicines/publications/essentialmedicines/en/.
16. Cea-Soriano L, Garcia Rodriguez LA, Machlitt A, Wallander MA. Use of prescription contraceptive methods in the UK general population: a primary care study. *BJOG* 2014; **121**(1): 53–60; discussion -1.
17. Superdrug/United Nations. Birth Control Around The World. 2017. https://onlinedoctor.superdrug.com/birth-control-around-the-world/.
18. Killick SR, Leary C, Trussell J, Guthrie KA. Sperm content of pre-ejaculatory fluid. *Hum Fertil (Camb)* 2011; **14**(1): 48–52.
19. National Health Service. Sexual and Reproductive Health Services - England 2016–17. https://digital.nhs.uk/catalogue/PUB30094.
20. Iversen L, Sivasubramaniam S, Lee AJ, Fielding S, Hannaford PC. Lifetime cancer risk and combined oral contraceptives: the Royal College of General Practitioners' Oral Contraception Study. *Am J Obstet Gynecol* 2017; **216**(6): 580 e1- e9.
21. Office For National Statistics. Cancer registration statistics, England. 2016. https://www.ons.gov.uk/peoplepopulationandcommunity/healthandsocialcare/conditionsanddiseases/bulletins/cancerregistrationstatisticsengland/2016.

22. Cancer Research UK. Cancer mortality statistics. 2017. http://www.cancerresearchuk.org/health-professional/cancer-statistics/mortality/common-cancers-compared.

23. Gallo MF, Lopez LM, Grimes DA, Carayon F, Schulz KF, Helmerhorst FM. Combination contraceptives: effects on weight. *Cochrane Database Syst Rev* 2014; (1): CD003987.

24. Mantha S, Karp R, Raghavan V, Terrin N, Bauer KA, Zwicker JI. Assessing the risk of venous thromboembolic events in women taking progestin-only contraception: a meta-analysis. *BMJ* 2012; **345**: e4944.

25. Lopez LM, Ramesh S, Chen M, et al. Progestin-only contraceptives: effects on weight. *Cochrane Database Syst Rev* 2016; (8): CD008815.

26. NICE. Clinical Knowledge Summary: Contraception – progestogen-only methods. 2017. https://cks.nice.org.uk/contraception-progestogen-only-methods.

27. Tyler KH, Zirwas MJ. Contraception and the dermatologist. *J Am Acad Dermatol* 2013; **68**(6): 1022–9.

28. Lopez LM, Chen M, Mullins Long S, Curtis KM, Helmerhorst FM. Steroidal contraceptives and bone fractures in women: evidence from observational studies. *Cochrane Database Syst Rev* 2015; (7): CD009849.

29. Hidalgo M, Bahamondes L, Perrotti M, Diaz J, Dantas-Monteiro C, Petta C. Bleeding patterns and clinical performance of the levonorgestrel-releasing intrauterine system (Mirena) up to two years. *Contraception* 2002; **65**(2): 129–32.

30. Lethaby A, Hussain M, Rishworth JR, Rees MC. Progesterone or progestogen-releasing intrauterine systems for heavy menstrual bleeding. *Cochrane Database Syst Rev* 2015; (4): CD002126.

31. Darney PD, Stuart GS, Thomas MA, Cwiak C, Olariu A, Creinin MD. Amenorrhea rates and predictors during 1 year of levonorgestrel 52 mg intrauterine system use. *Contraception* 2018; **97**(3): 210–4.

32. Gemzell-Danielsson K, Schellschmidt I, Apter D. A randomized, phase II study describing the efficacy, bleeding profile, and safety of two low-dose levonorgestrel-releasing intrauterine contraceptive systems and Mirena. *Fertil Steril* 2012; **97**(3): 616–22 e1-3.

33. Crosby RA, DiClemente RJ, Wingood GM, Lang D, Harrington KF. Value of consistent condom use: a study of sexually transmitted disease prevention among African American adolescent females. *Am J Public Health* 2003; **93**(6): 901–2.

34. Andrade AT, Pizarro Orchard E. Quantitative studies on menstrual blood loss in IUD users. *Contraception* 1987; **36**(1): 129–44.

35. Hubacher D, Chen PL, Park S. Side effects from the copper IUD: do they decrease over time? *Contraception* 2009; **79**(5): 356–62.
36. Duane M, Contreras A, Jensen ET, White A. The Performance of Fertility Awareness-based Method Apps Marketed to Avoid Pregnancy. *J Am Board Fam Med* 2016; **29**(4): 508–11.
37. Berglund Scherwitzl E, Gemzell Danielsson K, Sellberg JA, Scherwitzl R. Fertility awareness-based mobile application for contraception. *Eur J Contracept Reprod Health Care* 2016; **21**(3): 234–41.
38. Belker AM, Thomas AJ, Jr., Fuchs EF, Konnak JW, Sharlip ID. Results of 1,469 microsurgical vasectomy reversals by the Vasovasostomy Study Group. *J Urol* 1991; **145**(3): 505–11.
39. Barnhart KT, Schreiber CA. Return to fertility following discontinuation of oral contraceptives. *Fertil Steril* 2009; **91**(3): 659–63.
40. Glasier A. Implantable contraceptives for women: effectiveness, discontinuation rates, return of fertility, and outcome of pregnancies. *Contraception* 2002; **65**(1): 29–37.
41. Stoddard AM, Xu H, Madden T, Allsworth JE, Peipert JF. Fertility after intrauterine device removal: a pilot study. *Eur J Contracept Reprod Health Care* 2015; **20**(3): 223–30.
42. Jain J, Dutton C, Nicosia A, Wajszczuk C, Bode FR, Mishell DR, Jr. Pharmacokinetics, ovulation suppression and return to ovulation following a lower dose subcutaneous formulation of Depo-Provera. *Contraception* 2004; **70**(1): 11–8.
43. Skovlund CW, Morch LS, Kessing LV, Lidegaard O. Association of Hormonal Contraception With Depression. *JAMA Psychiatry* 2016; **73**(11): 1154–62.
44. Wirehn AB, Foldemo A, Josefsson A, Lindberg M. Use of hormonal contraceptives in relation to antidepressant therapy: A nationwide population-based study. *Eur J Contracept Reprod Health Care* 2010; **15**(1): 41–7.
45. Schaffir J, Worly BL, Gur TL. Combined hormonal contraception and its effects on mood: a critical review. *Eur J Contracept Reprod Health Care* 2016; **21**(5): 347–55.
46. Worly BL, Gur TL, Schaffir J. The relationship between progestin hormonal contraception and depression: a systematic review. *Contraception* 2018.
47. Duke JM, Sibbritt DW, Young AF. Is there an association between the use of oral contraception and depressive symptoms in young Australian women? *Contraception* 2007; **75**(1): 27–31.
48. Fergusson DM, Horwood LJ, Boden JM. Abortion and mental health disorders: evidence from a 30-year longitudinal study. *Br J Psychiatry* 2008; **193**(6): 444–51.

49. Biaggi A, Conroy S, Pawlby S, Pariante CM. Identifying the women at risk of antenatal anxiety and depression: A systematic review. *J Affect Disord* 2016; **191**: 62–77.
50. Wellings K, Jones KG, Mercer CH, et al. The prevalence of unplanned pregnancy and associated factors in Britain: findings from the third National Survey of Sexual Attitudes and Lifestyles (Natsal-3). *Lancet* 2013; **382**(9907): 1807–16.
51. Nappi RE, Lobo Abascal P, Mansour D, Rabe T, Shojai R, Emergency Contraception Study G. Use of and attitudes towards emergency contraception: a survey of women in five European countries. *Eur J Contracept Reprod Health Care* 2014; **19**(2): 93–101.
52. Glasier AF, Cameron ST, Fine PM, et al. Ulipristal acetate versus levonorgestrel for emergency contraception: a randomised non-inferiority trial and meta-analysis. *Lancet* 2010; **375**(9714): 555–62.
53. Marston C, Meltzer H, Majeed A. Impact on contraceptive practice of making emergency hormonal contraception available over the counter in Great Britain: repeated cross sectional surveys. *BMJ* 2005; **331**(7511): 271.
54. Cleland K, Zhu H, Goldstuck N, Cheng L, Trussell J. The efficacy of intrauterine devices for emergency contraception: a systematic review of 35 years of experience. *Hum Reprod* 2012; **27**(7): 1994–2000.
55. Department of Health and Social Care. Report on abortion statistics in England and Wales for 2016. 2017. https://www.gov.uk/government/statistics/report-on-abortion-statistics-in-england-and-wales-for-2016.
56. Livshits A, Machtinger R, David LB, Spira M, Moshe-Zahav A, Seidman DS. Ibuprofen and paracetamol for pain relief during medical abortion: a double-blind randomized controlled study. *Fertil Steril* 2009; **91**(5): 1877–80.
57. Halpern V, Raymond EG, Lopez LM. Repeated use of pre- and postcoital hormonal contraception for prevention of pregnancy. *Cochrane Database Syst Rev* 2014; (9): CD007595.
58. Macklon NS, Geraedts JP, Fauser BC. Conception to ongoing pregnancy: the 'black box' of early pregnancy loss. *Hum Reprod Update* 2002; **8**(4): 333–43.
59. Lohr PA, Fjerstad M, DeSilva U, Lyus R. Abortion: Clinical Review. *British Medical Journal* 2015; **348**: f7553.
60. Wilson E, Free C, Morris TP, et al. Internet-accessed sexually transmitted infection (e-STI) testing and results service: A randomised, single-blind, controlled trial. *PLoS Med* 2017; **14**(12): e1002479.

61. Sonnenberg P, Ison CA, Clifton S, et al. Epidemiology of Mycoplasma genitalium in British men and women aged 16–44 years: evidence from the third National Survey of Sexual Attitudes and Lifestyles (Natsal-3). *Int J Epidemiol* 2015; **44**(6): 1982–94.

62. Wiesenfeld HC, Manhart LE. Mycoplasma genitalium in Women: Current Knowledge and Research Priorities for This Recently Emerged Pathogen. *J Infect Dis* 2017; **216**(suppl_2): S389–S95.

63. Kingston M, French P, Higgins S, et al. UK national guidelines on the management of syphilis 2015. *Int J STD AIDS* 2016; **27**(6): 421–46.

64. Brunham RC, Gottlieb SL, Paavonen J. Pelvic inflammatory disease. *N Engl J Med* 2015; **372**(21): 2039–48.

65. Korostil IA, Ali H, Guy RJ, Donovan B, Law MG, Regan DG. Near elimination of genital warts in Australia predicted with extension of human papillomavirus vaccination to males. *Sex Transm Dis* 2013; **40**(11): 833–5.

66. Garland SM, Steben M. Genital herpes. *Best Pract Res Clin Obstet Gynaecol* 2014; **28**(7): 1098–110.

67. Cernik C, Gallina K, Brodell RT. The treatment of herpes simplex infections: an evidence-based review. *Arch Intern Med* 2008; **168**(11): 1137–44.

68. Public Health England. Towards elimination of HIV transmission, AIDS and HIV-related deaths in the UK 2017. https://assets. publishing.service.gov.uk/government/uploads/system/uploads/ attachment_data/file/675809/Towards_elimination_of_HIV_ transmission_AIDS_and_HIV_related_deaths_in_the_UK.pdf.

69. Antiretroviral Therapy Cohort C. Survival of HIV-positive patients starting antiretroviral therapy between 1996 and 2013: a collaborative analysis of cohort studies. *Lancet HIV* 2017; **4**(8): e349–e56.

70. Rodger AJ, Cambiano V, Bruun T, et al. Sexual Activity Without Condoms and Risk of HIV Transmission in Serodifferent Couples When the HIV-Positive Partner Is Using Suppressive Antiretroviral Therapy. *JAMA* 2016; **316**(2): 171–81.

71. Ballini A, Cantore S, Fatone L, et al. Transmission of nonviral sexually transmitted infections and oral sex. *J Sex Med* 2012; **9**(2): 372–84.

72. Chow EPF, Walker S, Hocking JS, et al. A multicentre double-blind randomised controlled trial evaluating the efficacy of daily use of antibacterial mouthwash against oropharyngeal gonorrhoea among men who have sex with men: the OMEGA (Oral Mouthwash use to Eradicate GonorrhoeA) study protocol. *BMC Infect Dis* 2017; **17**(1): 456.

73. Chow EP, Howden BP, Walker S, et al. Antiseptic mouthwash against pharyngeal Neisseria gonorrhoeae: a randomised

controlled trial and an in vitro study. *Sex Transm Infect* 2017; **93**(2): 88–93.

74. Giannaki M, Kakourou T, Theodoridou M, et al. Human papillomavirus (HPV) genotyping of cutaneous warts in Greek children. *Pediatr Dermatol* 2013; **30**(6): 730–5.

75. Davies S. The cervical smear test: does timing have an effect on sample adequacy? *Cytopathology* 2006; **17**(4): 182–6.

76. Petry KU, Horn J, Luyten A, Mikolajczyk RT. Punch biopsies shorten time to clearance of high-risk human papillomavirus infections of the uterine cervix. *BMC Cancer* 2018; **18**(1): 318.

77. Kyrgiou M, Mitra A, Arbyn M, et al. Fertility and early pregnancy outcomes after treatment for cervical intraepithelial neoplasia: systematic review and meta-analysis. *BMJ* 2014; **349**: g6192.

78. Joura EA, Giuliano AR, Iversen OE, et al. A 9-valent HPV vaccine against infection and intraepithelial neoplasia in women. *N Engl J Med* 2015; **372**(8): 711–23.

79. Mouchet J, Salvo F, Raschi E, et al. Human papillomavirus vaccine and demyelinating diseases-A systematic review and meta-analysis. *Pharmacol Res* 2018.

80. Pharmacovigilance Risk Assessment Committee (PRAC) of the European Medicines Agency. Assessment report. Review under Article 20 of Regulation (EC) No 726/2004, human papillomavirus (HPV) vaccines. EMA/762033/2015., 2015.

81. Drolet M, Benard E, Boily MC, et al. Population-level impact and herd effects following human papillomavirus vaccination programmes: a systematic review and meta-analysis. *Lancet Infect Dis* 2015; **15**(5): 565–80.

82. Landy R, Birke H, Castanon A, Sasieni P. Benefits and harms of cervical screening from age 20 years compared with screening from age 25 years. *Br J Cancer* 2014; **110**(7): 1841–6.

83. Kang WD, Choi HS, Kim SM. Is vaccination with quadrivalent HPV vaccine after loop electrosurgical excision procedure effective in preventing recurrence in patients with high-grade cervical intraepithelial neoplasia (CIN2-3)? *Gynecol Oncol* 2013; **130**(2): 264–8.

84. Garcia-Closas R, Castellsague X, Bosch X, Gonzalez CA. The role of diet and nutrition in cervical carcinogenesis: a review of recent evidence. *Int J Cancer* 2005; **117**(4): 629–37.

Part Four

1. Barnhart KT, Schreiber CA. Return to fertility following discontinuation of oral contraceptives. *Fertil Steril* 2009; **91**(3): 659–63.

2. Glasier A. Implantable contraceptives for women: effectiveness, discontinuation rates, return of fertility, and outcome of pregnancies. *Contraception* 2002; **65**(1): 29–37.

3. Stoddard AM, Xu H, Madden T, Allsworth JE, Peipert JF. Fertility after intrauterine device removal: a pilot study. *Eur J Contracept Reprod Health Care* 2015; **20**(3): 223–30.

4. Jain J, Dutton C, Nicosia A, Wajszczuk C, Bode FR, Mishell DR, Jr. Pharmacokinetics, ovulation suppression and return to ovulation following a lower dose subcutaneous formulation of Depo-Provera. *Contraception* 2004; **70**(1): 11–8.

5. Steiner AZ, Pritchard D, Stanczyk FZ, et al. Association Between Biomarkers of Ovarian Reserve and Infertility Among Older Women of Reproductive Age. *JAMA* 2017; **318**(14): 1367–76.

6. Birch Petersen K, Hvidman HW, Forman JL, et al. Ovarian reserve assessment in users of oral contraception seeking fertility advice on their reproductive lifespan. *Hum Reprod* 2015; **30**(10): 2364–75.

7. Qi X, Pang Y, Qiao J. The role of anti-Mullerian hormone in the pathogenesis and pathophysiological characteristics of polycystic ovary syndrome. *Eur J Obstet Gynecol Reprod Biol* 2016; **199**: 82–7.

8. Colombo B, Masarotto G. Daily fecundability: first results from a new data base. *Demogr Res* 2000; **3**: [39] p.

9. Manders M, McLindon L, Schulze B, Beckmann MM, Kremer JA, Farquhar C. Timed intercourse for couples trying to conceive. *Cochrane Database Syst Rev* 2015; (3): CD011345.

10. Levine H, Jorgensen N, Martino-Andrade A, et al. Temporal trends in sperm count: a systematic review and meta-regression analysis. *Hum Reprod Update* 2017; **23**(6): 646–59.

11. Kovac JR, Khanna A, Lipshultz LI. The effects of cigarette smoking on male fertility. *Postgrad Med* 2015; **127**(3): 338–41.

12. Ricci E, Al Beitawi S, Cipriani S, et al. Semen quality and alcohol intake: a systematic review and meta-analysis. *Reprod Biomed Online* 2017; **34**(1): 38–47.

13. Sallmen M, Sandler DP, Hoppin JA, Blair A, Baird DD. Reduced fertility among overweight and obese men. *Epidemiology* 2006; **17**(5): 520–3.

14. Grieger JA, Grzeskowiak LE, Bianco-Miotto T, et al. Pre-pregnancy fast food and fruit intake is associated with time to pregnancy. *Hum Reprod* 2018; **33**(6): 1063–70.

15. Karayiannis D, Kontogianni MD, Mendorou C, Douka L, Mastrominas M, Yiannakouris N. Association between adherence to the Mediterranean diet and semen quality parameters in male partners of couples attempting fertility. *Hum Reprod* 2017; **32**(1): 215–22.

16. Muscogiuri G, Palomba S, Lagana AS, Orio F. Current Insights Into Inositol Isoforms, Mediterranean and Ketogenic Diets for Polycystic Ovary Syndrome: From Bench to Bedside. *Curr Pharm Des* 2016; **22**(36): 5554–7.

17. Showell MG, Mackenzie-Proctor R, Jordan V, Hart RJ. Antioxidants for female subfertility. *Cochrane Database Syst Rev* 2017; **7**: CD007807.

18. Obeid R, Holzgreve W, Pietrzik K. Is 5-methyltetrahydrofolate an alternative to folic acid for the prevention of neural tube defects? *J Perinat Med* 2013; **41**(5): 469–83.

19. Gaskins AJ, Chavarro JE. Diet and fertility: a review. *Am J Obstet Gynecol* 2018; **218**(4): 379–89.

20. Garcia-Larsen V, Ierodiakonou D, Jarrold K, et al. Diet during pregnancy and infancy and risk of allergic or autoimmune disease: A systematic review and meta-analysis. *PLoS Med* 2018; **15**(2): e1002507.

21. Van Heertum K, Rossi B. Alcohol and fertility: how much is too much? *Fertil Res Pract* 2017; **3**: 10.

22. Lyngso J, Ramlau-Hansen CH, Bay B, Ingerslev HJ, Hulman A, Kesmodel US. Association between coffee or caffeine consumption and fecundity and fertility: a systematic review and dose-response meta-analysis. *Clin Epidemiol* 2017; **9**: 699–719.

23. Owe KM, Nystad W, Stigum H, Vangen S, Bo K. Exercise during pregnancy and risk of cesarean delivery in nulliparous women: a large population-based cohort study. *Am J Obstet Gynecol* 2016; **215**(6): 791 e1- e13.

24. King R, Dempsey M, Valentine KA. Measuring sperm backflow following female orgasm: a new method. *Socioaffect Neurosci Psychol* 2016; **6**: 31927.

25. Tanbo T, Fedorcsak P. Endometriosis-associated infertility: aspects of pathophysiological mechanisms and treatment options. *Acta Obstet Gynecol Scand* 2017; **96**(6): 659–67.

26. Brown J, Farquhar C. Endometriosis: an overview of Cochrane Reviews. *Cochrane Database Syst Rev* 2014; (3): CD009590.

27. Duffy JM, Arambage K, Correa FJ, et al. Laparoscopic surgery for endometriosis. *Cochrane Database Syst Rev* 2014; (4): CD011031.

28. Baird DD, Dunson DB, Hill MC, Cousins D, Schectman JM. High cumulative incidence of uterine leiomyoma in black and white women: ultrasound evidence. *Am J Obstet Gynecol* 2003; **188**(1): 100–7.

29. Cobo A, Garcia-Velasco JA, Coello A, Domingo J, Pellicer A, Remohi J. Oocyte vitrification as an efficient option for elective fertility preservation. *Fertil Steril* 2016; **105**(3): 755–64 e8.

30. Mesen TB, Mersereau JE, Kane JB, Steiner AZ. Optimal timing for elective egg freezing. *Fertil Steril* 2015; **103**(6): 1551-6 e1-4.

Part Five

1. Brown KF, Rumgay H, Dunlop C, et al. The fraction of cancer attributable to modifiable risk factors in England, Wales, Scotland, Northern Ireland, and the United Kingdom in 2015. *Br J Cancer* 2018; **118**(8): 1130–41.

2. Joseph DN, Whirledge S. Stress and the HPA Axis: Balancing Homeostasis and Fertility. *Int J Mol Sci* 2017; **18**(10).

3. Vanman EJ, Baker R, Tobin SJ. The burden of online friends: the effects of giving up Facebook on stress and well-being. *J Soc Psychol* 2018; **158**(4): 496–507.

4. Fenster L, Waller K, Chen J, et al. Psychological stress in the workplace and menstrual function. *Am J Epidemiol* 1999; **149**(2): 127–34.

5. Torner L. Actions of Prolactin in the Brain: From Physiological Adaptations to Stress and Neurogenesis to Psychopathology. *Front Endocrinol (Lausanne)* 2016; **7**: 25.

6. Wang L, Wang X, Wang W, et al. Stress and dysmenorrhoea: a population based prospective study. *Occup Environ Med* 2004; **61**(12): 1021–6.

7. Chen YT, Tenforde AS, Fredericson M. Update on stress fractures in female athletes: epidemiology, treatment, and prevention. *Curr Rev Musculoskelet Med* 2013; **6**(2): 173–81.

8. Jimena P, Castilla JA, Peran F, et al. Adrenal hormones in human follicular fluid. *Acta Endocrinol (Copenh)* 1992; **127**(5): 403–6.

9. Nargund VH. Effects of psychological stress on male fertility. *Nat Rev Urol* 2015; **12**(7): 373–82.

10. Frederiksen Y, Farver-Vestergaard I, Skovgard NG, Ingerslev HJ, Zachariae R. Efficacy of psychosocial interventions for psychological and pregnancy outcomes in infertile women and men: a systematic review and meta-analysis. *BMJ Open* 2015; **5**(1): e006592.

11. Akimoto-Gunther L, Bonfim-Mendonca Pde S, Takahachi G, et al. Highlights Regarding Host Predisposing Factors to Recurrent Vulvovaginal Candidiasis: Chronic Stress and Reduced Antioxidant Capacity. *PLoS One* 2016; **11**(7): e0158870.

12. Nansel TR, Riggs MA, Yu KF, Andrews WW, Schwebke JR, Klebanoff MA. The association of psychosocial stress and bacterial vaginosis in a longitudinal cohort. *Am J Obstet Gynecol* 2006; **194**(2): 381–6.

13. Cutter WJ, Norbury R, Murphy DG. Oestrogen, brain function, and neuropsychiatric disorders. *J Neurol Neurosurg Psychiatry* 2003; **74**(7): 837–40.

14. Nillni YI, Toufexis DJ, Rohan KJ. Anxiety sensitivity, the menstrual cycle, and panic disorder: a putative neuroendocrine

and psychological interaction. *Clin Psychol Rev* 2011; **31**(7): 1183–91.

15. Tiggemann M, Hayden S, Brown Z, Veldhuis J. The effect of Instagram "likes" on women's social comparison and body dissatisfaction. *Body Image* 2018; **26**: 90–7.

16. Gorczyca AM, Sjaarda LA, Mitchell EM, et al. Changes in macronutrient, micronutrient, and food group intakes throughout the menstrual cycle in healthy, premenopausal women. *Eur J Nutr* 2016; **55**(3): 1181–8.

17. Hildebrandt BA, Racine SE, Keel PK, et al. The effects of ovarian hormones and emotional eating on changes in weight preoccupation across the menstrual cycle. *Int J Eat Disord* 2015; **48**(5): 477–86.

18. Aune D, Giovannucci E, Boffetta P, et al. Fruit and vegetable intake and the risk of cardiovascular disease, total cancer and all-cause mortality-a systematic review and dose-response meta-analysis of prospective studies. *Int J Epidemiol* 2017; **46**(3): 1029–56.

19. Tavallaee M, Joffres MR, Corber SJ, Bayanzadeh M, Rad MM. The prevalence of menstrual pain and associated risk factors among Iranian women. *J Obstet Gynaecol Res* 2011; **37**(5): 442–51.

20. Parazzini F, Di Martino M, Candiani M, Vigano P. Dietary components and uterine leiomyomas: a review of published data. *Nutr Cancer* 2015; **67**(4): 569–79.

21. Harris HR, Eke AC, Chavarro JE, Missmer SA. Fruit and vegetable consumption and risk of endometriosis. *Hum Reprod* 2018; **33**(4): 715–27.

22. NHS Digital HaSCIC. Health Survey for England 2016; Fruit & Vegetables. 2016. http://healthsurvey.hscic.gov.uk/data-visualisation/data-visualisation/explore-the-trends/fruit-vegetables.aspx.

23. Zhao J, Lyu C, Gao J, et al. Dietary fat intake and endometrial cancer risk: A dose response meta-analysis. *Medicine (Baltimore)* 2016; **95**(27): e4121.

24. Qiu W, Lu H, Qi Y, Wang X. Dietary fat intake and ovarian cancer risk: a meta-analysis of epidemiological studies. *Oncotarget* 2016; **7**(24): 37390–406.

25. Thorning TK, Raben A, Tholstrup T, Soedamah-Muthu SS, Givens I, Astrup A. Milk and dairy products: good or bad for human health? An assessment of the totality of scientific evidence. *Food Nutr Res* 2016; **60**: 32527.

26. Chavarro JE, Rich-Edwards JW, Rosner B, Willett WC. A prospective study of dairy foods intake and anovulatory infertility. *Hum Reprod* 2007; **22**(5): 1340–7.

27. LaRosa CL, Quach KA, Koons K, et al. Consumption of dairy

in teenagers with and without acne. *J Am Acad Dermatol* 2016; **75**(2): 318–22.

28. Food Standards Agency and Public Health England. National Diet and Nutrition Survey (NDNS) 2018.

29. Baker JM, Al-Nakkash L, Herbst-Kralovetz MM. Estrogen-gut microbiome axis: Physiological and clinical implications. *Maturitas* 2017; **103**: 45–53.

30. Mueller NT, Duncan BB, Barreto SM, et al. Earlier age at menarche is associated with higher diabetes risk and cardiometabolic disease risk factors in Brazilian adults: Brazilian Longitudinal Study of Adult Health (ELSA-Brasil). *Cardiovasc Diabetol* 2014; **13**: 22.

31. Gong TT, Wu QJ, Vogtmann E, Lin B, Wang YL. Age at menarche and risk of ovarian cancer: a meta-analysis of epidemiological studies. *Int J Cancer* 2013; **132**(12): 2894–900.

32. Collaborative Group on Hormonal Factors in Breast C. Menarche, menopause, and breast cancer risk: individual participant meta-analysis, including 118 964 women with breast cancer from 117 epidemiological studies. *Lancet Oncol* 2012; **13**(11): 1141–51.

33. Mueller NT, Jacobs DR, Jr., MacLehose RF, et al. Consumption of caffeinated and artificially sweetened soft drinks is associated with risk of early menarche. *Am J Clin Nutr* 2015; **102**(3): 648–54.

34. Cheng G, Buyken AE, Shi L, et al. Beyond overweight: nutrition as an important lifestyle factor influencing timing of puberty. *Nutr Rev* 2012; **70**(3): 133–52.

35. Kastorini CM, Milionis HJ, Esposito K, Giugliano D, Goudevenos JA, Panagiotakos DB. The effect of Mediterranean diet on metabolic syndrome and its components: a meta-analysis of 50 studies and 534,906 individuals. *J Am Coll Cardiol* 2011; **57**(11): 1299–313.

36. Shai I, Schwarzfuchs D, Henkin Y, et al. Weight loss with a low-carbohydrate, Mediterranean, or low-fat diet. *N Engl J Med* 2008; **359**(3): 229–41.

37. Rogerson D. Vegan diets: practical advice for athletes and exercisers. *J Int Soc Sports Nutr* 2017; **14**: 36.

38. Harris HR, Chavarro JE, Malspeis S, Willett WC, Missmer SA. Dairy-food, calcium, magnesium, and vitamin D intake and endometriosis: a prospective cohort study. *Am J Epidemiol* 2013; **177**(5): 420–30.

39. Myung SK, Ju W, Choi HJ, Kim SC, Korean Meta-Analysis Study G. Soy intake and risk of endocrine-related gynaecological cancer: a meta-analysis. *BJOG* 2009; **116**(13): 1697–705.

40. Dong JY, Qin LQ. Soy isoflavones consumption and risk of breast cancer incidence or recurrence: a meta-analysis of prospective studies. *Breast Cancer Res Treat* 2011; **125**(2): 315–23.

41. Jamilian M, Asemi Z. The Effects of Soy Isoflavones on Metabolic Status of Patients With Polycystic Ovary Syndrome. *J Clin Endocrinol Metab* 2016; **101**(9): 3386–94.

42. Thoma ME, Klebanoff MA, Rovner AJ, et al. Bacterial vaginosis is associated with variation in dietary indices. *J Nutr* 2011; **141**(9): 1698–704.

43. Marco ML, Heeney D, Binda S, et al. Health benefits of fermented foods: microbiota and beyond. *Curr Opin Biotechnol* 2017; **44**: 94–102.

44. Public Health England. Health matters: getting every adult active every day. 2016.

45. Matthewman G, Lee A, Kaur JG, Daley AJ. Physical activity for primary dysmenorrhea: a systematic review and meta-analysis of randomized controlled trials. *Am J Obstet Gynecol* 2018.

46. Thomas RJ, Kenfield SA, Jimenez A. Exercise-induced biochemical changes and their potential influence on cancer: a scientific review. *Br J Sports Med* 2017; **51**(8): 640–4.

47. Boutcher SH. High-intensity intermittent exercise and fat loss. *J Obes* 2011; **2011**: 868305.

48. Almenning I, Rieber-Mohn A, Lundgren KM, Shetelig Lovvik T, Garnaes KK, Moholdt T. Effects of High Intensity Interval Training and Strength Training on Metabolic, Cardiovascular and Hormonal Outcomes in Women with Polycystic Ovary Syndrome: A Pilot Study. *PLoS One* 2015; **10**(9): e0138793.

49. Carvalhais A, Natal Jorge R, Bo K. Performing high-level sport is strongly associated with urinary incontinence in elite athletes: a comparative study of 372 elite female athletes and 372 controls. *Br J Sports Med* 2017.

50. Teixeira RV, Colla C, Sbruzzi G, Mallmann A, Paiva LL. Prevalence of urinary incontinence in female athletes: a systematic review with meta-analysis. *Int Urogynecol J* 2018.

51. Woodyard C. Exploring the therapeutic effects of yoga and its ability to increase quality of life. *Int J Yoga* 2011; **4**(2): 49–54.

52. Oates J. The Effect of Yoga on Menstrual Disorders: A Systematic Review. *J Altern Complement Med* 2017; **23**(6): 407–17.

53. Nidhi R, Padmalatha V, Nagarathna R, Amritanshu R. Effects of a holistic yoga program on endocrine parameters in adolescents with polycystic ovarian syndrome: a randomized controlled trial. *J Altern Complement Med* 2013; **19**(2): 153–60.

54. Oosthuyse T, Bosch AN. The effect of the menstrual cycle on exercise metabolism: implications for exercise performance in eumenorrhoeic women. *Sports Med* 2010; **40**(3): 207–27.

55. Sleep Council. The Great British Bedtime Report 2017. 2018. https://sleepcouncil.org.uk/sdm_downloads/the-great-british-bedtime-report-2017/.

56. Donga E, van Dijk M, van Dijk JG, et al. A single night of partial sleep deprivation induces insulin resistance in multiple metabolic pathways in healthy subjects. *J Clin Endocrinol Metab* 2010; **95**(6): 2963–8.

57. Romans SE, Kreindler D, Einstein G, Laredo S, Petrovic MJ, Stanley J. Sleep quality and the menstrual cycle. *Sleep Med* 2015; **16**(4): 489–95.

58. Webley GE, Leidenberger F. The circadian pattern of melatonin and its positive relationship with progesterone in women. *J Clin Endocrinol Metab* 1986; **63**(2): 323–8.

59. Jehan S, Auguste E, Hussain M, et al. Sleep and Premenstrual Syndrome. *J Sleep Med Disord* 2016; **3**(5).

60. Baker FC, Mitchell D, Driver HS. Oral contraceptives alter sleep and raise body temperature in young women. *Pflugers Arch* 2001; **442**(5): 729–37.

61. Poole R, Kennedy OJ, Roderick P, Fallowfield JA, Hayes PC, Parkes J. Coffee consumption and health: umbrella review of meta-analyses of multiple health outcomes. *BMJ* 2017; **359**: j5024.

62. Fenster L, Quale C, Waller K, et al. Caffeine consumption and menstrual function. *Am J Epidemiol* 1999; **149**(6): 550–7.

63. Whelan EA, Sandler DP, McConnaughey DR, Weinberg CR. Menstrual and reproductive characteristics and age at natural menopause. *Am J Epidemiol* 1990; **131**(4): 625–32.

64. Evans SM, Levin FR. Response to alcohol in women: role of the menstrual cycle and a family history of alcoholism. *Drug Alcohol Depend* 2011; **114**(1): 18–30.

65. van der Schuur WA, Baumgartner SE, Sumter SR. Social Media Use, Social Media Stress, and Sleep: Examining Cross-Sectional and Longitudinal Relationships in Adolescents. *Health Commun* 2018: 1–8.

66. Li C, Kee YH, Lam LS. Effect of Brief Mindfulness Induction on University Athletes' Sleep Quality Following Night Training. *Front Psychol* 2018; **9**: 508.

67. Baron KG, Abbott S, Jao N, Manalo N, Mullen R. Orthosomnia: Are Some Patients Taking the Quantified Self Too Far? *J Clin Sleep Med* 2017; **13**(2): 351–4.

Index

light: blue light 233, 236
  and sleep 229
LLETZ treatment, cervix 146–8
luteal phase, menstrual cycle
    30–1, 190, 229–30, 234

magnesium 194
male fertility 162–3, 175, 192
male sterilisation 103
medication: and absent periods
    49–51
  medical abortion 116–17
  and the Pill 107–8
meditation 194–5, 235
Mediterranean diet 163–4,
    207
melatonin 229, 230, 233, 235–6
menopause 31
  premature 44, 182, 231
menstrual cups 31–3
menstrual cycle 26–31, 75
  alcohol and 234
  appetite and 200
  caffeine and 231
  and exercise 216, 220–1
  fertility-awareness
    contraception 101, 102
  irregularity 40
  and sleep 227
  stress and 189–91
  tracking 35
mental health: abortion and 119
  hormones and 195–6
  oral contraception and 106–7
  social media and 196
metabolism 199–200, 205
metformin 50
metronidazole 128
microbiome: gut 205, 209
  vagina 77, 209
mifepristone 116, 117
mindfulness 236
minerals 208
Mirena coil 97–9
miscarriage 112, 167, 190
misoprostol 116, 117–18
mobile phones 102–3, 233, 236
mons pubis 2

morning-after pill (MAP) 109–10,
    111, 119–20
Mound of Venus 2
mucus, cervical 76, 95, 97
muscles: exercise 199–200,
    215–17, 220
  pelvic-floor 5, 7, 206, 217–18,
    224
Mycoplasma genitalium 128, 130

Nabothian follicles 13–14
noradrenaline 46, 189

oestrogen 15
  and absent periods 42, 44
  and constipation 205–6
  contraceptive ring 95–6
  and exercise 220
  and fat tissue 199
  heavy periods 57, 59
  lack of 52
  menstrual cycle 30–1
  oral contraception 89, 94
  premenstrual syndrome 65
  sleep and 229, 230–1
  soy-rich foods 209
  stress and 191–2, 195–6
Omega-3 fatty acids 165–7
oral contraception 12, 89–95
  combined oral contraceptive
    pill (COCP) 89–94, 104, 106,
    107
  and depression 106–7
  and discharges 75
  failure to work 107–8
  'fake periods' 36
  and future pregnancy 105
  health benefits 90–1
  irregular and absent periods
    43–4, 49–50
  and period pain 62
  progesterone-only pill (POP) 95,
    104, 106, 107
  side effects 91–4
  stopping 159
  stopping periods 37
oral sex 126, 132, 135–6
orgasm 10, 170